DYSLEXIA

VISUALLY DEAF?
AUDITORY BLIND?

GARY CHEVIN

authorHOUSE®

AuthorHouse™ UK Ltd.
500 Avebury Boulevard
Central Milton Keynes, MK9 2BE
www.authorhouse.co.uk
Phone: 08001974150

First published by AuthorHouse 3/5/2009

ISBN: 978-1-4389-6319-8 (sc)
ISBN: 978-1-4389-6320-4 (hc)

Printed in the United States of America
Bloomington, Indiana

This book is printed on acid-free paper.

Professor Rod Nicolson Dean of psychology University of Sheffield

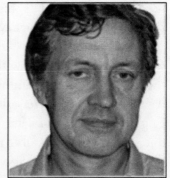

I have known Gary Chevin for four years now, and have had the pleasure of working closely with him in attempting to investigate his conviction that dyslexic adults (and children) suffer from a lack of 'inner voice' – the language of thought. When most of us think, it is in some form akin to abbreviated language. Having learned to speak out loud in their first two years, children spend another four years or so learning to 'internalise' the speech, that is to be able to 'talk in their head', and this forms the basis of thought. Quite how this happens, and what format inner speech takes remains a mystery even now – in my view one of the most important issues for cognitive psychology. When I quizzed Gary about his own inner speech, he said that he had had none until recently when he trained himself to develop a rudimentary form. When he thinks, he 'sees a blur of images, overlapping and displacing each other, but no words'. I could not imagine how anyone can cope without inner speech, and we have spent the past few years developing tests for inner speech, so as to identify how widespread this problem is. Gary is convinced that the problem is particularly associated with dyslexia and with attention deficit.

The process of learning to read 'scaffolds' the internalisation process by encouraging the reader to read silently, though normally some inner speech is in place before silent reading occurs. Nonetheless, if a child has not developed an effective inner speech before he or she is taught to read, this may well have an adverse effect on the learning process. It is surprising that this key issue has been ignored in the science of reading instruction. If Gary is right, it would have a major impact on education theory and practice.

A lack of inner speech would also lead to a difficulty in remembering what was said. Imagine a child is being told off by a teacher or parent. The teacher makes a remark that the child needs to qualify or correct. Lack of inner speech prevents retention of the response, so the child has to 'use it or lose it'. There is no opportunity to wait until it's

1

the child's turn to speak. Hence the child interrupts, causing further aggravation, or listens dumbly, unable to comment or clear himself (or herself). Gary considers this analysis provides a key insight into the apparently disrespectful behaviour of young offenders.

A further important concept that Gary introduces is that of 'confusion'. We are all familiar with this state. Imagine not being able to recall the name of a good friend when having to introduce them, or perhaps trying to hold a conversation in a noisy café with several non-native English speakers. For some reason the brain is working inefficiently or one just can't take in all that's happening. It's as though the brain gets filled with 'noise' that stops normal memory processes working. One normally has to wait until the confusion clears In Gary's view, confusion is the typical state for a dyslexic children in a classroom, with the effect that their learning processes become very significantly impaired. I believe that confusion is also an important concept that has been under-researched.

The third key contribution made by Gary is in his efforts to overcome the difficulties caused by lack of inner speech and by confusion. Naturally he has hit upon a visual strategy for remembering information. His mnemonic strategy based on linking the appearance of a letter (or number) to its name or meaning is a particularly powerful method, of value whether or not one's inner speech is strong, but of particular value when inner speech is weak.

Gary is strongly dyslexic. He has high creativity and very weak reading ability. I encouraged Gary to write this book because I felt he had much to contribute. Consider the difficulties he faced: he writes by dictating to 'speech to text' software. He reads the text via text-to-speech software. His weak inner speech means that he cannot remember what he has just read. It is therefore not surprising that the book lacks structure in some parts, and that the organisation is limited. The strength of the book is its very immediacy. Gary 'tells it like he saw it', with an emotional rawness, a creativity, and a directness that I found very engaging.

It's book to be read as quickly as possible, from beginning to end. There is something in this book for everyone. Inspiration for an individual with dyslexia and insight for us all.

Rod Nicolsom
Professor of Psychology, University of Sheffield

Professor Angela Fawcett, researcher into dyslexia

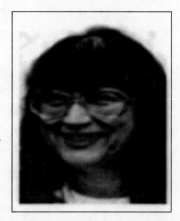

I have been researching into dyslexia for over 20 years,since our son Matthew-was diagnosed with dyslexia at the unu-sually early age of 5. I was driven bymy need to find out more about the causes of dyslexia and how it impacted onthe lives of people with dyslexia and their families. Over this period, I havemet many people with dyslexia, and became aware that my husband David and mostof his family were dyslexic. The author of this book, Gary Chevin, who came toa conference on dyslexia to challenge our academic preconceptions, may well bethe most colourful character I have met in the dyslexia world. Gary hasdeveloped his own theory of dyslexia, based on his recognition that he lackedan inner voice which others seemed to use to help them in reading. Garychallenged us to work with him to research these ideas and our research to datesuggests that young children in the early stages of reading acquisition mayin-deed be dependent on this inner voice in order to read. In this book, Garypresents a compelling story in his own words of his struggle to achieveliteracy, and allows us a rare insight into the spectrum of diffi-culties whichcharacterise dyslexia, far removed from the reading prob-lems which have beenthe major focus of research in the area. I recom-mend this book to all those whoseek a deeper understanding of what it means to be a dyslexic adult.

Angela Fawcett

David Fawcett,successful adult dyslexic, retired business manager for major global corporation

I picked up Gary's book with some trepidation, because as an adult withdyslexia,it is years since I have read a complete book. For one of the raretimes in my life, I found this to be a book which I could not put down. I readthe whole book in just two weeks and was fascinated by the insight that Garyhas into the whole condition of dyslexia, an insight which few so-calledexperts in the field would share. Not only did I find his whole storycompelling, but I feel strongly that it should be published in as near the sameformat as presented to me in draft. Any attempt in 'correction' or attempt at'clarity' would to be my mind be a grave mistake, because the text as it standsdemonstrates the immense effort undertaken by Gary in producing such a book. Whilst appreciating and understanding his sentiments and the difficulties thecondition has presented for him,. However,this book should be compulsory reading for all educational psychologists and teachers since they will all encounter people like Gary and myself, and it would help if they understood that the condition involves more than just reading and spelling

David Fawcett

Dr Gerald Lombard Chartered Psychologist

Gary is a life-long student and researcher without formal qualifications or the rigour of academia but with the understanding and creativity of an innovator. I have listened to his theories based on empirical research from respected scientists, read his contributions and watched the application of his eclectic approach with teenage students who were unable to read - and I do believe he is worth listening to, to enable some young people with written communication who could benefit from his approach. I am most impressed that this is a cognitive motivational approach rather than being purely repetitive/functional or programme-based. I hope a wider ranging research project will follow.

Dr Gerald Lombard
Chartered Psychologist

CONTENTS

You have purchased this book because you have an interest in dyslexia you maybe a teacher a parent or you may be dyslexic some people believe dyslexia is a gift I'm not too sure about that my experiences have not been a gift to me it was one of the most frustrating areas of my life underachieving failing and embarrassment you may have read other books on dyslexia you may have an understanding but the question I must ask, do you truly understand how I feel I know quite a lot about blind people but I really do not understand how they feel and the challenges they face .

I remember somebody telling me a story you can learn how to ride a bike out of a book you then can teach how to ride a bike but the question is can you ride a bike no you learn how to ride by experience and this is how dyslexia is a lifetime of experiences I am going to try to explain dyslexia in this book keeping it simple and easy to follow I hope you enjoy.

Dyslexia from a dyslexic's point of view

What is dyslexia? It seems like an easy enough question, what should have an easy enough answer. But this is not the case. For years, specialists have researched this area; they used to believe that dyslexic people had brain damage, or nerve damage, ear and eye problems. Dyslexia has been researched four over 100 years one of the early researchers in dyslexia   Huey (**1908**) recognized that inner   cognitive supermodel as an **internal** feedback route from **speech** .But what does that mean when I hear academics talk about dyslexia it is like listening to a foreign language . Dyslexia is not a result of brain damage, or nerve damage, ear or eye conditions .The specialists tell us, that there are many different forms of dyslexia, but how can this help the students, parents, and teachers. Some dyslexic students can read fairly well, there problem is, they don't understand what they read, other students find it virtually impossible to read at all. So what is dyslexia? What is the true meaning of dyslexia? It is only my belief. But I believe that dyslexia is a different way of thinking, a self-created condition created at a very early age. But how does this work? As a dyslexic person I often wondered, what was the difference between a dyslexic person and a none dyslexic person. It is widely believed, that people think in two different ways, verbal thought, and picture thought. Verbal thought means, thinking in the sound of speech, the fastest that anyone could think in verbal thought, is 150 words per minute .This is one area what shows a difference between dyslexics, and none dyslexics. As a dyslexic, I very rarely use verbal thought, and as I looked at this area, it became clear that many more dyslexics felt the same .Picture thinking is a natural way of thinking we do it from a very early age but picture thinking is so much faster than verbal thought is governed by words. It is very hard to understand a picture way of thinking at times, it happens so quickly you are not even aware of it .In the period when dyslexia is being developed, a person is a non-verbal thinker, this is a person who thinks in pictures. When you are using a picture way of thinking, you are thinking in pictures this process is many times faster than verbal thought. How can this way of thinking restrict the way the dyslexic students learn? When reading, the dyslexic students must verbalise what they are reading, if they don't, their understanding is extremely reduced. Why? Many Dyslexics have no or a very fragmented internal monologue. I believe, the internal monologue is apart of verbal thinking. The dyslexic did not develop a verbal way of thinking, it is a developmental process, the dyslexic preferred a picture way of thinking, that is much faster and clearer .The problem is, when you choose a picture way of thinking, your thinking far to quickly, and you are not developing a step by step linear approach, what you need in a learning environment Also, another process as not been developed its reason and logic, reason and logic are language based, an internal process what goes with the internal monologue. I needed to know what a none dyslexic person was doing internally when reading , I was shocked to find out that when reading internally they could hear clearly , I found this virtually impossible to do. This is how I came up with the phrase visually deaf , when reading internally your eyes become your ears, what you see you hear internally, think about this ?.Most dyslexics find it virtually impossible to do, so they are visually deaf .I wanted to know what a none dyslexic person, was doing when they were spelling. Shut your eyes, and then get somebody to give you a spelling, what do you see? Do you see the word internally? I have never seen a word internally; this makes me auditory blind, the inability to see what I hear when spelling .Think about this? No or very little internal monologue! Not using a step by step linear approach, not using conventional reason and logic. Visually deaf and auditory blind, thinking far too quickly. Now you can see why, we have so many problems, in the academic environment. All because, we preferred a pictorial way of thinking.

!welcome to my dyslexic world

WHAT IS DYSLEXIA?

The word 'dyslexia' comes from the Greek and means 'difficulty with words'.**Definition:** Dyslexia is a specific learning difficulty which mainly affects the development of literacy and language related skills. It is likely to be present at birth and to be lifelong in its effects. It is characterized by difficulties with phonological processing, rapid naming, working memory, processing speed, and the automatic development of skills that may not match up to an individual's other cognitive abilities. It tends to be resistant to conventional teaching methods, but its effects can be mitigated by appropriately specific intervention, including the application of information technology and supportive counseling.But what does this mean it leaves me no wiser surely after 100 years somebody should know. What is Dyslexia to me yes problems with reading and writing but there's so much more the embarrassment I went through on a day-to-day basis mass confusion the feeling of hopelessness the feeling of being alone the depression having problems understanding what people say missing appointments getting the days wrong the sheer frustration of not being self sufficient the inability to learn spelling you learn one you learn another one after three you forgotten the first one looking at text on a book and not knowing what it says the feeling of failure the way that people treat you they do not know what to do and come up with their own interpretations what can offend you they believe they know best but they don't and the problems I have with forgetting things so frustrating nobody truly understands .When I look at a page of text I can see the letters not jumping about or falling off the page I know the names of each letter I can even tell you what sounds them letters make but my problem is putting them letters together to make a word it is like climbing a mounting with outer rope and blindfolded and the funny thing is it is them smaller words this what cause the most problems .

Gary, why did you write this book? My motivation to write this book was to let people know of what we had found and try to give an insight of how a dyslexic person feels from school, 1 to work, and beyond, helping parents, teachers,, and even dyslexic people to understand and try to alleviate the confusion and frustration they face on a day-to-day basis. I would also like to thank Professor Rod Nicolson, for his patients understanding and belief, as an academic he has an open mind and does not have the terrible condition of ego and Professor Angela Fawcett .Dyslexic people suffer with confusion but their parents and teachers suffer too the problem with dyslexia so many theories nearly everyone different as chalk and cheese.

THEORIES
Breath test can identify dyslexia.

Cause of dyslexia narrowed down to single chromosome.

The discovery of a hereditary link to dyslexia.

Intensive training can 'jump-start' dyslexics' brains.

Balance exercises can help pupil performance.

Research backs controversial DDAT approach to dyslexia.

So many theories academics disagreeing with each other dyslexics confused parents and teachers confused my question was why . So what is dyslexia we are led to believe it is hearing problems problems with the eyes nerve damage brain development but is it in my opinion dyslexia is problems with internalising sound the ability to internalise sound is important when reading you are internalising the words on the page manipulating sound mass confusion the dyslexic student suffers confusion on a day-to-day basis confusion restricts the students ability to learn thinking too quickly the dyslexic students have not slowed down the way that they think they think in pictures running at a phenomenal speed when you learn to read your thinking in words picture thinking is so much faster not developing a linear way of thinking the dyslexic students have not developed linear thought the ability to follow information in order .

With the theory comes a solution there are hundreds of solutions to cure dyslexia, I have met many people who believe the solution I met one parent who truly believed in fish oil her Son had been taking it for 12 months she Said it improved his concentration and helped him with reading, I couldn't say she was wrong she had strong belief. I met another parent who truly believed her son's improvement came from wearing colored lenses her belief was great. I have met parents who believe in movement therapy, all of these parents had something it was belief.But how could this be, they were all different it could be hearing problems, eye problems, or other problems, the list goes on, this led me to believe no one truly understood this condition that is dyslexia.I have met many people who follow strict regimes following systems they believe in, they also think they have the cure, but how can this be they are so different. How are they helping, maybe it is the belief that helps dyslexics, they suffer with confusion, and self-limiting beliefs, maybe the belief in the system allows them to overcome their confusion and self limited belief.So what do we need to do, where colour lenses, one eye covered by a patch, drinking fish oil, and hopping on one leg, if we do all of this surely we will cure dyslexia .So when you're reading this keep an open mind we are trying to find something all dyslexics have in common, by doing this we are getting close to what dyslexia really is, is this the true definition?....

So Gary... In that section is it really that confusing? Yes, I have met hundreds of parents, you see it in their faces they look lost and even the teachers they are looking for an answer that no one can give them. Are there really that many different theories from all over the world? Yes there have I hear it all of the time" breakthrough" " cure" another group of researchers has discovered what dyslexia is.But how many of them have got it right, how this condition can change so rapidly. I understand with technology new doors open but how confident are they. Recently I heard dyslexia the myth, one professor said there was no such thing as dyslexia how could this be I have been told for the past 48 years I am dyslexic, does his theory say I have been lied to, or the teaching methods were not good Enough or Gary wasn't bright enough not dyslexic just a bit slow, how does this make me feel. Another Professors new theory.Enough or Gary wasn't bright enough not dyslexic just a bit slow, how does this make me feel. Another Professors new theory... May be I Haven't I been trying hard enough, or is he saying I do not exist as a dyslexic I wish they would make up their minds.I decided to contact this Professor, his name was Julian Elliot, I e-mailed him he responded I asked him if he had really thought about what he was saying and the implication it could have on the dyslexic community, how would teachers interpret his theory it would make them think dyslexia doesn't exist what about the students at school and the implications his theory would have.When you make such profound statements you should always think about the implications, specially if you're in a privileged position like Professor Elliott, I heard of another breakthrough "cure" once again using this terminology this surely does not help when you say" you have the cure" this leads people to believe dyslexia is a disease and it is not, I wish people would think more about what they are saying because dyslexia is a condition that affects millions of people they need positive help not statements just for publicity .I was contacted by a dyslexic woman who was very angry she did a March in London with a placard saying there's no such thing as an academic she was very upset with what Mr. Elliott comments, he carried on with his opinion on dyslexia I told him I could not see the point of it and the damage it was creating he ignored this and carried on I don't truly believe he truly understands the condition of dyslexia he Just thinks it is reading, writing, and spelling, but any one who truly understands this they know it is so much more.

Gary... Do you really think what Professor Elliott said really influenced what people thought? Yes... Since Professor Elliot, made his statement I have heard people talk about dyslexia in a negative way.

DOES EVERY ONE START OUT DYSLEXIC?

One of the questions I asked myself when we are children nobody begins with the ability to read and write everybody starts from the same place the place, I call dyslexia and as the Child learns and progresses they move out of the state of dyslexia and become readers but the Child who does not master reading will stay there everybody starts out dyslexic in my opinion.By the age of 40 Gary had a reading age of seven years all I wanted to do is to learn one spelling and remember it but this was not as easy as it sounds I had problems with the building blocks of literacy I had to design new building blocks what would allow

me to work with them I finally did it created my own alphabet and learned how to spell but even more retain it .As I start writing this book I'm trying to remember my experiences as a child something I find hard to do my memories are very weak it was a very painful experience they seem to be locked away them early memories of childhood,

I really don't think people truly understand the pain this experience created, the mind is a funny thing when something is painful it locks your memories away.

THE BIGGEST LIE IN THE WORLD

What do I mean the biggest lie in the world? When I was a child, I was extremely close to my sister; there was exactly two years between us   we were more like twins. I remember the worst day of my life, it was the day my sister started school , myself and my mother took her their , we left her at the gates , I looked at her and started to cry . That day was like a year, I remember waiting for her to come home. When we met her, she seemed different she was still my sister, but she seemed different. I asked her what was the school like, she said great and fantastic. I couldn't weight to start school, if my sister said it was great it must be.

It was soon my turn, I remember that day butterflies in my stomach, nervous and scared. The first day, it wasn't what I expected. I remember the teacher she was young but she never smiled, things were getting bad to worse,

THE DAY OF THE LOST BOOK

the day of the lost book, The teacher who never smiled, was more angry than I had ever seen her, where is the book she shouted no one will leave this room Intel it is found but where had the book gone everybody was looking for it under tables in draws but nobody could find it she got angrier and angrier her face went read her eyes went wide where is the book some children began to cry she went into the cloakroom and shook everybody's coat mine was next she shook it and the book fell out she picked it up and marched over to me shaking it in the hair you had the book Chevin I was so scared my head drooped and I looked at the floor Chevin look at me she shouted I looked up as she grabbed my shirt shaking me violently I was so scared I wet myself it ran down my leg and made a puddle on the floor go to the corner of the room and look at the corner and do not turnaround it was terrible my sister said it was brilliant but it was not I hated it and I hated books why did she tell me such a massive lie I was only six .

Gary. . The section on starting school many children go through the same experience as you surly? , yes they do but they are not all dyslexic are they. School is a scary experience for children however, those children soon got used to it and the work I did at school never made sense to me.

What were the signs? Umm! Well Gary kept on losing his book every time it was reading at school and Gary's book went missing again.

I remember the teacher who used to help me with reading she was an extremely old lady with thick rimmed glasses she had problems with her dentures they used to float around her mouth she never really helped in fact she gave me the answers I didn't even ask.

I remember the look on the faces of the teachers they looked confused, you see Gary wasn't a slow learner but he just could not master literacy they tried it just wouldn't go in.At this time I realized I was different and the other students realized it too children have a natural ability to home in on something different it is not thought about they just do it some people say it is bullying, it is just what children do and this is when I became a fighter if somebody said something to me I would fight back children can be so hurtful.

School got harder I further and further behind my friends were now reading but

Gary had no idea how to use these things what they called letters.

Gary did you really feel that different? Yes when you're sitting in a room and you feel you're the only one who can't do it, it makes you feel different and you turn to fighting I must have been eight or nine when I realized if you hit them they didn't treat you like a fool it was my defence.

MY QUANTUM LEAP

I must have been nine years old school was getting difficult I didn't want to go how can you get out of school, its illness, when you're poorly you don't have to go, but I was not ill, so what were the other options. I remember that morning walking to school past the old church, on the far side to the church there was a high wall that dropped into the entry behind the terraced houses; I stood on the wall looking down umm! If I jump and hurt my leg I won't have to go to school this was my decision but I was scared, oh! what happens if I really injured myself not just hurt my leg I could cripple myself I stood there looking shall I shan't I.

My mouth was very dry what shall I do it was nearly time to go to school another day of sheer hell another day of embarrassment another day of feeling stupid I looked down then jumped I saw the floor rushing towards me then I hit it I heard something crack tremendous pain shot up my leg but a feeling of satisfaction I had done it no school today in fact I was off school for five weeks this a major accomplishment what worries me what length would I have taken to get out of school injuring myself the length I went through to get out of school I could easily of crippled myself but I felt I had no other option how many other children felt their options were limited that they would feel they had no other option.

Did my parents know what I was doing no nobody truly understood what I was going through it was a lonely place for the young Gary and it really didn't improve .

The quantum leap this was extreme **Gary?** Yes it was extreme but I felt I had known other option I felt alone there was no one to talk too and explain how I felt. How far would you have gone? I don't really know students have committed suicide would I have done this I don't know I suppose it was an option if things didn't improve .

From a very early age Gary knew he was different but one thing was in my favour I was good at sport Cricket, football, and swimming, I swam for my city when I was at school doing sport I was as good as any one around me this made me feel good. This is the problem for the dyslexic child they feel different not in a good way you just know your different. The years of my primary school were not so bad it's when I started the secondary school everything changed. I always had a problem with school. Over the last few years I got used to it but now I'm going to a different school where the children are big and everything will be different For some apparent reason the teachers were different the compassion was not there that I had found in the primary these teachers were harder they roared louder it could have been years and years of teaching children it had worn them down they had lost the reason why they started teaching I don't blame them however, my fear returned. In this place, they expected every child to read and write and know their time tables and God help you if you didn't know corporal punishment today we can't even imagine an adult beating the Child with a stick I remember this treatment if your work wasn't good enough they beat you if you couldn't spell the words they asked they beat you coming in late they beat you I was beat on a regular basis I remember that came long and thin one teacher used to pickle it in water he could bend it in a circle and when it hit you it felt like a bite them cruel days of corporal punishment .I remember the stream of teachers all believing they were going to master my problem and teach me how to read, after one month their enthusiasm was there but after seven and eight months the enthusiasm faded one year later they disappeared and another new teacher was there telling me that they would teach me how to read, everyone failed but what they really didn't understand is the damage they were doing they felt like a failure because they could not teach me however they felt even worse they had failed "once you had". When you have failed hundreds of times on your reading your self confidence and self-esteem is in pieces.

THE GIANT

His name was Mr. Sandywell he must have been 6.7" tall 20 stones in weight he was recognised as the hardest caner in the school every one was scared of him, when he hit, you stayed hit, he didn't talk he roared you could hear him All over the school other teachers would send you to him for punishment I believe, he enjoyed it.

CHEVIN, you are the boy who cannot read I will teach you he roared I had no choice, come to me Monday lunchtime and we will begin. I remember that first day I was terrified the first lesson was over come next week he roared, this went on for several months did I improve no I could see it in his eyes he was not succeeding and this affected him it was quite obvious he liked to win but with Gary he felt the failure isn't that strange I was not improving but he felt a failure probably that is what teachers feel when they cannot help a student to succeed they feel like they have failed but they haven't, they have been to university they are the teacher but just imagine it, what you have been trained to do and you can't. After seven months it ended he never spoke of it again and I forgot it too. **Gary** was secondary school that different? yes you see in primary School they are teaching you how to read and write preparing you for secondary school when you get their they expect you to have the ability to read and write if you cannot it messes up their systems you become a problem and no one likes problems .

Gary how did this make you feel ? I must be honest not too good it felt like I was on conveyor belt it didn't help in any way in fact it made me feel worse it drew attention to myself special lessons Chevin the other children said .

STRENGTHS

A lot of people focus on the weaknesses of Dyslexia, and they don't even understand those. They don't even consider the strengths of Dyslexia, and That means they even have less understanding. Dyslexics are visual, imaginative, lateral, global, intuitive, picture thinkers. People talk about dyslexic strengths what does that mean something you're good at? yes my own strengths are I was very creative, artistic, at school but what else I suppose I'm pretty good at problem-solving how do I do it?I have a problem I see it then forget it, maybe the next day or the next week the answer comes to me I just see it, many times I don't know how I got their if you asked me how did I find a solution I wouldn't know. This was one of the strangest ways I learnt, I was classed as a slow learner yes, with literacy, and mathematics, but out of this field I am Extremely quick at learning. My work was in the building industry one-day I was sitting in a JCB digger I sat at the controls and began to dig without thinking then I realised what I was doing I had never been taught how to do this but I could do it without thinking many years I had been in Jobs with the drivers never asking how to do it but subconsciously I was watching and learning, you see I learn extremely quickly without thinking about it subconscious learning.Dyslexic strengths have been observed by specialists this is a list of a few of the strengths.

· Creativity
· Thinking laterally and making connections
· being able to see the 'big picture'
· Good visual spatial skills and being able to think easily in 3D
· Problem solving skills
· Good verbal skills

And this is a list of people who used these unique skills.

   · Albert Einstein
   · Tom Cruise
   · Cher
   · Walt Disney
   · Thomas Edison
   · General George Patton
   · Nelson Rockefeller
   · Pablo Picasso
   · Hans Christian Anderson
   · Leonardo da Vinci
   · Richard Branson
   · Sir Winston Churchill
   · Gustavo Flaubert
   · Steven Spielberg
   · President Kennedy

When I realised Albert Einstein was dyslexic this gave me a feeling of satisfaction one of the most intelligent men in the last century struggled like I did but his work clearly showed his strengths.Einstein showed language impairments at a very young age. His speech was severely delayed. He was late with speech he began to talk at the age of three, and had trouble with language throughout elementary school. a parent meeting, the Headmaster told Einstein's parents that he did not have the ability to be a successful. He recommended that Einstein attend a trade school. In fact, his teachers thought he was borderline retarded.Young Albert did not listen to them. Instead, he moved to a different type of school. This school de-emphasized rote memorization. Unlike his old school, they stressed creative thinking and hands-on learning. Young Albert's academic performance improved dramatically. Which of these skills was Einstein using when he came up with his theory?

· Creativity
· Thinking laterally and making connections
· Being able to see the 'big picture'
· Good visual spatial skills and being able to think easily in 3D
· Problem solving skills
· Good verbal skills

May be all of them.

Winston Churchill - This statesman could be called academically Disadvantage. He failed grade eight, did terrible in maths and generally hated school. He failed his entrance exams two or three times into military Academy It wasn't until these two men broke away from school and the negative way that they were taught they were not allowed to show their strengths development in the academic straitjacket it is only when they left school they started to develop them to the degree they did that allowed them to become the geniuses, they were .We must look at to- day... Bill Gates he was one of the richest men in the world he developed and created Microsoft. Richard Branson one of the richest men in the UK created Virgin.

RICHARD BRANSON...

Richard Branson, founder and chairman of London-based Virgin Group, didn't breeze through school. In fact, school was something of a nightmare for him. His scores on standardized tests were dismal, pointing to a dismal future. He was embarrassed by his dyslexia and found his education becoming more and more difficult. He felt as if he had been written off How ever, his educators failed to detect his true gifts. His ability to connect with people on a personal level, an intuitive sense of people, was not detected until a frustrated Richard Branson started a student newspaper with fellow student Jonny Gems. The incredible success of the Student was but the start of a richly diverse and successful career. Despite the difficulties and challenges posed by his dyslexia, by focusing on his inner talents, Richard Branson successfully overcame his difficulties. From his first taste of success and believing in himself, Richard Branson never looked back.Alan sugar, an entrepreneur worth millions how many of these men use their dyslexic strengths to become who they are, was their highly developed creativity responsible for their success? But how many of the potentials, your Einstein's, Churchill's, are destroyed by the education system not helping their strengths to grow but to be destroyed. A staggering 35% of US entrepreneurs suffer from dyslexia, compared to 20% in the UK, a groundbreaking study by Julie Logan, Professor of Entrepreneurship at Cass Business School, reveals

Gary do you think the business world misses out because their knowledge on dyslexic strengths is unknown? Yes if the business world truly understood how dyslexics really think and the benefits they could bring to business they would be seeking them out but the truth is they end up on scrap heaps and this is a great mistake.

CONFUSION

I was confused all the way through the primary School but here my confusion became impounded I had no idea what they were talking about I just couldn't work it out

A DAY IN SCHOOL

34 students sat down on a Monday morning it was an English lesson I sat at the back of the classroom trying not too draw attention to myself the teacher wrote on the board it was a lesson on Shakespeare he talked about what was going on then he asked the students to copy from the board. Their books opened they picked up their pens and started to copy from the board I sat there not knowing what it said not knowing what it meant, I began to copy one letter at a time it was like time slowed down one letter then another letter word after word, I didn't know what I was writing down it was so monotonous, then the teacher said stop… I looked at the page I had done under a paragraph the letters were different sizes and running up and down the page the student to my left had completed a full-page oh.. What was the point what have I learnt, another day of confusion frustration there does not seem a point to it?

CONFUSION THE DOWNWARD SPIRAL

From a very early age I had met confusion it has lived with me nearly all of my life but how damaging is confusion occurs when a person's brain is not functioning properly. People experiencing confusion have problems remembering, paying attention speaking, thinking, and reasoning, and understanding accurately what is going on around them. They may also find that their usual sleep patterns are disturbed. Confusion is the inability to think with your usual speed or clarity. When confused, you have difficulty focusing your attention and may feel disoriented Confusion interferes with your ability to make decisions.

CONFUSION AND DYSLEXIA

I have seen hundreds of different approaches to help dyslexia and a lot of them work, they are all different from the traditional methods .There are other wonderful methods apart from what the system said you must follow.

Could it be that these traditional   methods are not helping the person with their literacy problems, but other methods are helping with confusion, the person is confused and by using other methods it alleviates the confusion that allows the person to improve with their literacy? If one method was used to alleviate the problems we could say this is the correct way but they are so diverse and this is where the problem is. One organisation says if you follow our system you will be cured just do this for 10 minutes a day for 12 months but what we should ask what is it doing they believe it is strengthening our brain but is it? I believe it is alleviating the confusion that allows the student to learn.

When the students attend these programmes it would be so much better if we could test the level of confusion they were suffering and after they have gone through this programme we could retest them and see if their level of confusion has dropped however, that has not been tested. People say dyslexia is different for each person I disagree the difference is how the Person handles confusion if we watch three people with the same problem and the problem creates confusion, we would see three different ways of handling it people are different.

And this is where the problem is, each academic has his theory and from this the approach is developed from brain, eyes, nervous system, the list goes on but one thing is certain…. with all the dyslexic people I see confusion, it is always there in one form or another confusion the crippling condition that restricts the students from their learning.Astronauts and other people who voyage into the unknown suffer from similar Symptoms, we could say they are based on confusion and disorientation. Information was found that astronauts were suffering from dyslexia type symptoms when returning to earth and polar expedition they suffered similar symptoms. In one case a person was asked what the capital of France they could not answer is it's experiencing these extreme conditions that caused confusion and disorientation.Knowing this it should give us an insight on how the Child perceives the unknown experiences of learning, could we put these experiences in the same level as space exploration maybe it is an unknown factor that creates confusion and disorientation the symptoms are similar affecting reading memory processing created through confusion and disorientation many times I remember a teacher explaining to me I could see their mouth moving but could not hear the words and if I did it was like they were speaking in a foreign language I would nod my head like I understood but the truth is I didn't I was experiencing mass confusion by this time there had been many years of confusion no one understood the damage it was doing I'd become used to it, was part of my life it became normal to be confused . If somebody else would have experienced what I was going through it would had probably made them quite ill this degree of confusion is extremely Damaging for the young child but no one knows the true degree of confusion the child is suffering.

DIFFERENT STAGES OF DYSLEXIA THE CONDITION

From severe to moderate what does that mean? I hear people say he is a bit dyslexic how does that work? I have a friend named Chris he did two years in university studying law a very difficult subject but Chris was dyslexic people would say he was a little bit dyslexic .When Chris reads he must read it four or five times to get any form of understanding and then he forgets a lot, how does he do it, well when reading he skips words, if Chris was reading this, he would be skip reading. You see Chris leaves words out completely we could say up to 60% of the information he does not read and the other 40% he could forget a great deal, his condition is not just a bit dyslexic in my opinion it is just as bad as not being able to read at all.As Chris is reading what happens is, he sees the first word that he is familiar with he then moves onto the next word this word creates confusion because he doesn't like confusion so he skips another word then he goes to the next word what is familiar to the previous words he then moves on the next three or four words he knows but the next three words creates confusion.Because he does not like confusion he skips it is the confusion that makes him skips the words he has trained himself to body swerve confusion.He is now in his thirties he has been using this technique for many years he does not even think about it is automatic it is subconscious as he reads he skips the words that creates confusion he is not even aware of it Michael is classed a severe dyslexic nearly all the words he has problems with his confusion starts straightaway the first word would be alien to him the confusion begins he Tries to push to the next word but this creates confusion he does not understand what he is reading and the confusion is devastating. They both suffer with confusion the confusion they experience will be Devastating in their understanding they will both be disadvantaged in the academic world. So knowing this confusion and how damaging confusion is why do we leave the child in this awful state? We! allowed this confusion to take over, learning becomes an impossibility but the problem is, the child becomes used to it subconsciously they do not like this feeling but after a period of time when it is missing it makes them feel strange, Confusion is a state of brain disfunction, also referred to as delirium. Confusion may range from mild—including slight forgetfulness, and inability to concentrate, to severe changes in a person's behaviour, personality and consciousness. Confusion is often reversible,

LOST IN THE DARK HOLE

Nearly everyone has experienced confusion once in their life maybe when you are learning how to drive can you remember it how did it make you feel? Nothing will go in you are hot and sweaty it did not matter how hard you tried it just would not go in. Imagine nearly every day of your life you experienced confusion. Reading is something most people do every day just imagine reading created the same confusion as when you are learning to drive how would that feel? Could you cope with it? This feeling is what people feel who have problems with literacy. When you're confused it is a natural instinct to try to get out of it you will do anything to get out of it but what happens if you can't

how do you handle this my confusion was crippling it felt like I was falling down a dark hole with no help. Dyslexia should be called Disconfusion because the main characteristic is confusion it is the confusion that restricts the learning, I believe if we could alleviate the confusion learning will be more natural.

CONFUSION AND SCHOOL

How does it occur? The child begins to learn how to speak it is learning through names, pictures, we learn like who is our mother and father its by what they look like your mother points to the cat and says cat black-and-white with long whiskers when she says cat You know the picture your language is learnt by what you see by the age of seven you've mastered your language.Your first days at school the teacher writes on the board three letters C A T and says CAT the confusion begins in your mind you see the picture of the black and white cat but she is pointing to three letters and says cat the word is CAT, whatever way you look at it you cannot see the cat the confusion begins.

So each new word gives you a picture that you learnt from your parents but the teacher is saying something different. I now have to put my trust in a person I do not know that is the teacher. Who do I believe of course a child believes their parents, in your mind you see your house but the letter H O U S E gives you nothing but more confusion? The problem we have is changing the picture into the word e g, you have a picture of a cat you place the word cat above the picture CONFUSION you are aware of the picture of a cat however, the word cat looks nothing like the picture of a cat and learning to put the word to the picture came naturally to us when we were learning how to speak. But now we expect the Child to change the way they have been learning since the age of three or so the confusion this creates which can damage the child for the rest of their lives if you do not alleviate the confusion.But how many educators are aware of the degree of the child's confusion.Their problems began with changing the picture to the written word something that simple has created their problems could it be possible that a large percentage of learning difficulties today in our schools are created by the child getting confused and not helping the child to alleviate it . But why do certain people have problems with this? It could it be the way they are thinking like a genetic influence, it is believed that people think in two ways picture, thought, and verbal, could the picture thinker be a person who has a strong tendency to develop picture thought to a higher degree have this problem. Do we have two separate modes of thinking and one becomes our primary mode and if you prefer the picture mode as your primary mode could this be where the problem is. The answer is YES and the verbal thinker is the person who does not develop picture thinking to this degree has no problem changing the words to a picture because they prefer verbal thought as their primary mode of thinking.

The problem with this degree of confusion is it can create problems later in life. A large percentage of people who suffer with dyslexia have depression and anxiety problems, many of them take prescription drugs also use alcohol trying to escape from their problems what were created many years previous from their confusion.

Gary the section on confusion do you really think confusion is one of the major influences what creates dyslexia? Yes… confusion is one of the major influences in the creation of dyslexia. Do you think schools look at the problem of confusion? I don't think they truly understand how damaging confusion is. I think there should be a bigger emphasis on the problem when a student gets confused learning is virtually impossible.

THE SILENT BULLY

In my middle years in secondary school I needed to change, this is when I met my first bully I remember him well along tall gangly youth he saw my weakness and homes in on it I was frightened not knowing what to do this went on for months when you're in this state there are two things you can do run, or fight, I began to run trying to find a way out but it was very difficult. This only compounded my problems and made it worse as I began to bob school running away from the bully, un-till I got caught, hear is another Problem through not going school, my parents punished me, the school punished me, and the bully punished me.Where does it end"suicide" is it a way out? Yes it crossed my mind.

THE DAY THE BLOOD RAN

It was a Monday morning just like any other Monday at school I hated it, but I was still there. It was late afternoon I was on the playground when the bully started again I don't know why but something happened inside me like a switch turning on he came towards me poking me in the chest from nowhere My hand connected with his face and his nose exploded blood splattered everywhere it was like slow motion as he fell to the ground whimpering and crying. All of a sudden I saw him different not this big tall gangly youth but a baby that's all. Things changed straight away the other children wanted to be with me wanted to know my name I had slayed the dragon I felt like a hero I'd changed what I was doing instead of running I fought back .Was that the answer to your problems if your attacked in any way was it fight back was that what you did?

THE INVISIBLE BULLY

But there was another bully who made me feel just as bad it would send terror through my soul I had two choices run or fight but this bully was different yes I was scared the feeling is just the same but this bully was endorsed by the teachers, this bully was the teacher's friends but this bully was invisible no one could see him but he was there how do you fight an invisible bully, who do you fight the teachers, the people, who endorsed him Yes fight the teachers they are just as bad as the bully.What did he look like what did he sound like I will tell you his name WORDS yes WORDS..... My invisible bully was WORDS.... they'd made me feel just the same as the tall gangly youth but how do you fight WORDS...They were everywhere in each classroom on every wall taunting me there was no escape in fact this bully was the worst what do you do run or fight but who do you fight the teachers, and then you get expelled they are not even aware why you are angry they are not even aware of this bully,, we hear of children being bullied at school committing suicide every one is looking out for it but the silent bully they're not aware of. I suffered for years and years of being bullied by WORDS... At the time you are not aware of it maybe you're too young but the feelings are the same as somebody bulllying you, how many children today are being bullied by WORDS... I must make people aware of the invisible bully of my childhood. I must be honest looking back on them days I don't know how I got through it. I hear people say schooldays the best days of their lives not for Gary these days were the worst.

Gary was the bullying that bad? Yes I experienced bullying from another student this was bad but if I am honest the bullying I experienced from WORDS... Was the worst it felt just the same but it was endorsed by the teachers I truly believe they were not aware of this but how many children today feel bullied in the same way it concerns me

The problem was I was in the bottom class after examinations Gary came bottom except in Art, and PE Gary came top, the crazy thing was Gary knew he was the cleverest in the class and the other students knew it too I used to think I wish I was stupid then I could except the fact that I was a slow learner but when you know you are the cleverest this is where the damage is Confusion, that was damaging but now we have frustration you know you're the cleverest but they treat you like a fool you haven't even got past Janet and John, the basic book that a Primary School child can read. Now you're 15 yrs old, different teaches really thought they were helping me, but I had been trying for years and years, even with special help nothing worked, it never made a difference I was totally confused and now to add on to my confusion it brought on frustration. In my final year at secondary school, I decided to stop going and developed an art for truancy and guess what? I was good at it, I never got caught I would get up in the morning and go to school my parents thought when they had gone to work I went to school. I came home went to my sister's room and with her makeup I created bruises all over my arm then made a sling and went out. One-day the Head Teacher saw me outside school when really I Hould have been in doing my school work, she asked me what was wrong I showed her my arm and she was so sympathetic I became really good at this .Through playing Truancy I forgot and neglected my art work, something I regret, yes! I got a pass, on three pieces of work, there should have been five However, and they passed me on three. My art teacher saw something in me and tried her best to encourage me to go to art College and study art; she even got her husband to visit me. He was a Lecturer at the Art college, they begged me to go but I didn't, if its one thing I regret it is not going, but you see in my mind College was like school and I'd had enough .

Gary that must have been extremely difficult knowing you was the brightest in your class? I don't want to sound arrogant but it was true, it is a well-known fact a large percentage of the dyslexic community are above-average but this is the problem, we have the intelligence to analyse our situation and this is damaging, even now I sit in front of civil servants, and teachers, I just know I have as much overall intelligence than them **Gary** tells me of your feelings on your final day at school? The happiest day of my school life was the final day; yes it was all over no more school the silent bully would leave me alone there would be no more sitting in that classroom totally confused not knowing what was going on, I counted down the days.

During the last week I didn't miss one-day, I got there on time and smiled all the while they were giving me my leaving certificate, and at four o'clock it was all over. I went out into the school yard and set my leaving certificate on fire and watched it burn, the smoke rising Upto the sky it was over no more school ever again the feeling was fantastic But what was the damage? What had it done to Gary,I had 11 years of hell, no one truly realised what I had been through all of the confusion the frustration, the anger, sometimes even cruelty the Teachers shouting at me, punishing me, for something I could not do. All this that I went through had damaged me, there was no doubt about that, in fact it felt like Child abuse, you can't get away from it, if you truly analysed my experiences of my school life you would be totally shocked, and you would have stopped it. No one believes in child abuse but how can a Teacher shout and punish you for something that is not your fault it's cruel. If you could imagine serving a prison term and counting each day of your sentence the day you will become free, that was school for me, I can truly say there is not one good memory that I can give to you. Many dyslexics are never tested for dyslexia I have been tested three times throughout my life the severity has always been the same as I read it I cannot believe it is talking about me it seems so damning .

GARY'S DYSLEXIA STATEMENT

Mr Chevin has a memory of experiencing significant learning difficulties throughout his statutory schooling period. He received remedial teaching. He left secondary school with a formal qualification in Art. Mr Chevin entered the building industry. However, he suffered a back injury and therefore no longer works

Mr Chevin reports a range of learning difficulties within the areas of communication, organisation, memory and concentration, literacy, orientation, maths, and co-ordination and dexterity.

Throughout my assessment, I noted that Mr Chevin had significant difficulties with word retrieval and mispronounced a range of words. The latter reflects underlying difficulties with phonological processingMr Chevin was assessed at the Dyslexia Institute (now Dyslexia Action) by my professional colleague, Mrs Stockley in March 2000. She concluded that …*(Gary) is a person with average general ability who is under achieving in reading, spelling and writing. His basic reading skills and spelling are well below average. The level of underachievement in spelling and writing is statistically significant at the 1% level… Gary is also well below average when processing material where a measurement of speed is involved, such as the Hedderly Sentence Completion Test. Gary shows a particular strength in his visual-spatial skills… The performance on this occasion show a pattern of strengths and weaknesses consistent with dyslexia …His scores place him in the F (Very Severe) Category on the Dyslexia Index, which measures the severity of the condition on a scale from A (no signs) to F (very severe).*

Mr Chevin's scores also indicate that his working memory capabilities lie within the extremely low range and at a percentile of 2. Working memory refers to the ability to "work on" information retained within the short-term memory store.Mr Chevin's ability to process low-grade visual information at speed, as measured by the WAIS III[UK] Processing Speed Index lies within the average range and at a percentile of 39.The above scores indicate that Mr Chevin has an extremely irregular profile of cognitive abilities, typically found within the dyslexic population. His main cognitive ability weakness resides within the working memory channels) Attainments in Core Literacy SkillsMr Chevin's single word recognition skills as tested by the (WIAT II [UK]) Word Reading subtest are at a percentile of less than 0.1.Mr Chevin's spelling skills as tested by the WRAT 4 are at a percentile of less than 0.1.Mr Chevin's ability to decode nonsense words are at a percentile level of 2. Nonsense word tests are used to establish the degree of a client's knowledge of phoneme (letter sounds)-grapheme (letters) links.The above three tests span the age equivalent range of 5 years 8 months and 6 years 4 months. It must be stressed that age equivalent scores are relatively unreliable and are extrapolated from normative data relevant to the tests' standardisation on children. It is my opinion that Mr Chevin has dyslexia of a very severe nature. The dyslexia is characterised by extremely delayed literacy skills levels, word retrieval and phonological processing difficulties, and a very weak working memory base. My findings concur with those reported by Mrs Stockley, specialist teacher.

It is my opinion that Mr Chevin would be perceived as 'disabled' according to the Disability Act 1995/2004 in that his dyslexia is severe enough to have a significant detrimental impact on his day-to-day living circumstances.I also believe that Mr Chevin would be regarded as "mentally vulnerable[1]" in an interview situation because he may not understand the significance of what is said, of questions or of their replies. Mr Chevin will forget large proportions of information put to him in the short term and/or be confused by this information. Most severely dyslexic people experience these sorts of difficulties. Some severely dyslexic people also become confused, anxious, troubled, etc. in stressful situations that load heavily on their dyslexia.It should be noted that Mr Chevin has normal verbal inductive reasoning capabilities as indicated by his scores on the Similarities WAIS III[UK] Scale. His long-term memory for retention of general knowledge is also normal as indicated by his score on the InformationMr Chevin's score on the WRAT 4 Sentence Comprehension scale was at a percentile of 0.1. This test measures a client's ability to understand the meaning of a written sentence.On a similar test, the Vernon Warden (Revised), Mr Chevin scored at a percentile level

STARTING WORK

My first job was working with a construction company doing all the maintenance on factories, I was offered an apprenticeship to become a bricklayer doing one day a week at College, when I got there I thought it would be beneficial but I had no problem with the practical side but then the invisible bully came back I had to do the theory there he was again taunting me I thought I had left him behind at school but no! he was also in college, the lecturer did not know what to do, so they decided practical bricklaying and then practical plumbing leaving out the theory, then they realised this could not be done I had to do my theory, they tried but nothing worked the WORD bully was back in the end I had to leave.

Gary this must have been terrible you wanted to learn a trade and the restrictions were their again? Yes I'm extremely good at learning things using my hands but I had to do the theory, back then there was no help for people with dyslexia, and it has changed, however, in my opinion not enough.

You see dyslexia doesn't only affect you at school, it affects your life, No qualifications, and now No trade, I was so depressed I believed I was the only dyslexic person in the world, I had never met another person with dyslexia, was I the only person with this crippling confusing problem called dyslexia…At this time I was suffering with my nerves I went into bouts of depression not knowing why, the depression would last for 3 to 4 months then it would disappear but deep down I knew it would return. This carried on for the next 10 years, I was just 25 yrs of age and then I had a massive attack what totally crippled me, I did not know what to do I had lived with fear most of my life but this was something that I had never experienced before I suffered with massive panic attack, I was totally out of control, you see I have a very vivid imagination dyslexic's have that, and when you're being creative it is beneficial however, it can be a double edged sword it can also work against you. Have you ever experienced fear so crippling you have problems with breathing, disorientation, confused, palpitations, stomach conditions, the list went on. I finally went to see the doctor and begged him for help, he gave me tranquillisers, he prescribed me Ativan… I had to take 3 a day, they did work and they helped me to find reality again, my fears subsided however, I did not feel right, an appointment was made to see a Psychiatrist I went to the hospital and waited for 1hr then I only saw him for 15 minutes I made another appointment for the next month I went back again this went on for 4months. I noticed the same people in the waiting room every time I went back, it might have been my imagination but they seem to getting worse not better All of these people looked like they were deteriorating, was I? so the next appointment I said thank you I feel better now, I did not want to be like them poor people so I decided not to go again and I never went back A degree of normality came back into my life I wasn't right, but, I could now go back to work you see I had just got married my wife did not know anything about what was going on so I had to go to work and try to fit in where I left off, However, I carried on taking these tranquillisers for the next 15 years I control the fear by carrying one with me if I had it in my pocket I felt safe.

What created my problems, could it have been than 11 years of hell living with confusion frustration bottling it up, and then it exploded like a volcano very hard to prove but looking at the facts it is possible. The only problem was Gary had been taking tranquillisers for over 15 years and I had become addicted to them another problem tranquilliser addiction   Dyslexia affects you in so many ways yes, you have problems with reading, writing, and maths but there are underlined problems, your self esteem is nonexistent, your confidence is shattered and now you know confusion lives with you. During the 15 years of being on medication I continued to work in the construction industry I was self-employed its very common with dyslexic people we find it hard to work for someone, I still had the problems but now I could hide them.

Gary a lot of people have suffered with depression and we know it is crippling how did you cope? It took maybe 6 or 7 years to come to terms with it after going through the traditional methods I met a lady who practised hypnosis this was very beneficial I learnt a lot from this I was still taking Tranquillisers living with fear but I felt I had begun to sort out my life it probably took 20 years to rectify it. **Gary** do you really think your problems were created by your school experience? Oh! Without a doubt, the degree of pressure I suffered would have created these problems and the anxiety year after year there's nothing else I can think of.

THE DAY I STOOD FOR PRIME MINISTER

You're probably thinking what Gary means by this. Well In 2005 in my City there was a local election and I ran for elected Mayor, a very responsible position, I thought yes I can do something with this City, Education for one thing, its very poor on Education plus it creates crime, because of the lack ofEducation there is also lot of unemployment because the industry has gone, there are no more Pottery firms or Coal mining or Steel Works I believed I could do something about it, the only problem was Gary decided to do this 10 weeks before the election, know where near enough time typical dyslexic, it has to be done NOW!...So I went on the election campaign I was not affiliated to any party I was independent I was focusing on Education and Disability and Senior Citizens I had invested everything I had, it cost me £10,000 I chose not tell my wife about the cost and I went for it . "She did find out though wives do oh dear "I visited Senior Citizen Centres knocked on doors, gave out balloons in my local City Centres went on the radio I was in the newspaper, I was very busy But you see Gary was a busy fool not enough thought running around like headless chicken yes, I understood the failure in Education and yes me Understood, disability problems but that was not enough .However, I did gain 5000 votes not bad for 10 weeks work. But I had £10,000 less than what I started out with, but I thought I could do something about our City I really believed I could of, but do I regret it no, it was an experience and I think that's what life is about a combination of experiences .I think what really attracted me to be a councillor, was that no one asks me are you qualified, you don't need qualifications to do hold this position this was one area where I stood an equal playing field every other area for every job they always ask me what are your qualifications but to be a counsellor you do not need them. When Tony Blair was Prime Minister of the United Kingdom his deputy prime minister was John Prescott he had a terrible time at school he failed his 11[plus] in fact, Mr Prescott has dyslexia…

In 1999 I had to finish work in the construction industry due to a injury I received early in my career the doctor advised me to find alternative employment and that is what I tried to do but I soon realised that at 40 years of age Gary was unemployable, I could not work in the construction industry I could not work if I had to lift and carry due to the severity of my injury plus the problems with my dyslexia as my reading age was seven years all other prospects needed literacy. What do you do when all your opportunities have disappeared my anxiety returned I was extremely depressed, I had two children and the house to run with very little finances to do it, your life is made up of events good and bad but what you need is a little bit of luck something that some how went against me. The next 18 months I was lost, not knowing what I could do, it has always been hard nothing seemed to come easily, but now the only way I could make money had disappeared what you do.

Gary how did you cope with what was happening? This was probably one of the worst experiences in my adult life you see I have always worked from England to Europe always knowing how I was going to create my income but now I was lost from £50,000 pa to income support this was a body blow and nobody could help me

FINDING OUT ABOUT THE SECRET

I decided once again to revisit reading I decided to try again this time to be successful to become a reader to prove to myself I could do it,   I needed it without it I had no future .The first month I started to read my wife helped me, the first page it was like stumbling through a dense forest everything feeling strange nothing felt familiar I completed the first paragraph but I did not know what I had read as I Look at the words what do I see? I see a combination of letters I know what each letter says but there's nothing after that. I must try to explain how it feels as I'm looking at the letters I recognise the letter **C** and the next letter is **O** followed by **M** then **B** So what do I see **COMB.** then add an **I** then followed by **O** then a **N** then an **A** ending with **I** then **O** then **N** but what does that say I have **lost** the **first sound** the **middle sound** and just have the **end sound I O N** put it all together you have the word **COMBINATION** as I am going through this I can feel the confusion growing in this state nothing makes sense.The more I try the harder it gets mistake after mistake, my self confidence and self belief is nonexistent, how many times must the average person fail before giving up maybe 3 times maybe 9 times maybe 30 times, I do not think the average person would try 30 times to try and do what they know they can not,   and not give up, how e.g. the word **COMBINATION....** when you are a reader you automatically internalise what you read when you are reading and I'm sure that'   but how do you do that, how do you get the words into your head and remember them internally   was this a secret that no one had told me how to do it? .Was I now suffering with self-limiting beliefs I had failed for all them years so do I now believe" it is totally impossible"   not only to read but now do it in my head

Gary do you think you will ever learn how to read? if I am honest NO… What I do know is you have to except the way you are, to move on. I've never met another dyslexic who has truly mastered it I have however, met people who have improved but they are still dyslexia

Theories of dyslexia What I found out

After 12 months I decided I must find out what is dyslexia why do I have it why does it stop me reading and can it be cured. ?. The dyslexic brain struggles to read because even small distractions can throw it off, according to a new model of dyslexia emerging from a group of recent studies. The studies contradict an influential, 30-year-old theory that blamed dyslexia on a neural deficit in processing the fast sounds of language. Instead, the studies suggest that children with dyslexia have bad filters for irrelevant data. As a result, they struggle to form solid mental categories for identifying letters and word. It has been commonly agreed that developmental dyslexia in different languages has a common biological origin: a dysfunction of left posterior temporal brain regions dealing with phonological processes I soon realised there was hundreds of theories on the subject so many and so different but they all believed their own theory how could this help all the Academics with different answers the Brain the Ear the Eyes, the list went on in fact this made me feel worse.

Gary how did you feel when you learnt about all these theories? so confused I believed somebody would have the answer all I saw was Academic disagreeing with each other and in many cases sounding ridiculous. I remember being at the British Dyslexia Association's conference five different Academics presented their opinions everyone different, I remember thinking if this room was full of dyslexics 50% of them would commit suicide Being told that they had a disease and the other 50% would Lynch the Academics for what they said under developed brain it was unbelievable it made us sound terrible.

Catching the secret

It was a Saturday afternoon Midsummer my wife was sitting in the garden reading the Saturday Newspaper to herself I was watching her reading but I noticed she was not moving her mouth when reading I asked, what are you doing she looked at me strange I'm reading, but you are not moving your mouth she replied I'm reading in my head, what does that sound like it sounds like my voice she said, just like your voice I said yes she replied.I was shocked when reading I must move my mouth and hear what I'm saying this concept of talking in your head was alien to me does everybody do this I asked her, yes of cause . I have two dyslexic children I asked my daughter can you hear your voice in your head when reading no! I asked my son he could not hear his voice inside his head also, I believed I had found something different over the next 18 months. I travelled around the UK meeting dyslexics my question to them was can you hear yourself internally when you are reading 90% of them said NO... could this have something to do with their inability to learn how to read correctly? Was their any other differences? I asked my wife as she is a reader questions about reading I found out when she was reading but even more when she was spelling she could see the word internally, she followed it through her mind something else I could not do, as I can't see words, letters, or anything to do with words "internally" I can see visual images quite easily but letters and words I just cannot see them could this be another part of my problem .

Gary how did it feel when you discovered the lack of internal speech? It took a few days to register, but it was a Eureka moment I had found something that all dyslexics have in common .

INNER SPEECH

I had discovered people who suffer with dyslexia they have not developed inner speech something that is lacking, everything started to make sense my poor memory skills that come from that inner voice, the mother asks the Child go to your room and bring me your towel, dirty clothes,, your school shoes, your School uniform and your PE kit that's 6 items his Mother has asked him to bring although the child heard his mother say this, its fallen out of mind he has forgot maybe two or three things that his Mother had asked him to get, if he had developed the "internal speech" he would have remembered, as he would have repeated it in his mind but because internal speech was lacking he forgot half of what his Mother asked. When the child looks at the words on the page he hears what they say internally he is following a running commentary it allows him to understand it, process it, and use it again.But the Child who has not developed internal speech will not have the same process going on he will look at the page see the words but will have no internal prompt to help him he knows what the letters are but putting them together internally is nonexistent .There was a problem with internal speech but could the person have a speech problem what had developed from an early age with verbalise speech what affected their development of internal speech ? .

INNER SPEECH IN THE LITERATURE

Dyslexia Signs:
Late Talking or Immature Speech

Research has revealed a dramatic link between the abnormal development of spoken language and learning disabilities such as dyslexia

Can the speech problems be visible, at a very early age could the Child show the symptoms but they are missed, and when speech goes inward the problems are compounded verbal speech was not developed correctly and internal speech was very poor . What types of speech and language disorders affect school-age children? Children may experience one or more of the following disorders: **speech sound disorders** – (difficulty pronouncing sounds) **language disorders** – (difficulty understanding what they hear as well as expressing themselves with words) **cognitive-communication disorders** – (difficulty with thinking skills including perception, memory, awareness, reasoning, judgment, intellect and imagination) **stuttering (fluency) disorders** – (interruption of the flow of speech that may include hesitations, repetitions, prolongations of sounds or words) **voice disorders** – (quality of voice that may include hoarseness, nasality, volume (too loud or soft)

DO SPEECH-LANGUAGE DISORDERS AFFECT LEARNING?

Speech and language skills are essential to academic success and learning. Language is the basis of communication. Reading, writing, gesturing, listening, and speaking are all forms of language. Learning takes place through the process of communication. The ability to communicate with peers and adults in the educational setting is essential for a student to succeed in school How may a speech-language disorder affect school performance Children with communication disorders frequently do not perform at grade level. They may struggle with reading, have difficulty understanding and   expressing language, misunderstand social cues, avoid attending school, show poor judgment, and have difficulty with tests.Difficulty in learning to listen, speak, read, or write can result from problems in language development. Problems can occur in the production, comprehension, and awareness of language sounds, syllables, words, sentences, and conversation. Individuals with reading and writing problems also may have trouble using language to communicate, think, and learn. In order to learn, a person must be able to store something that he has perceived and decoded, so that he will be able to recall this information at a later stage. It is the ability to recall to memory or to remember that makes learning possible. Memory is one of the foundational skills of learning that is of special importance in the so-called learning subjects at school or university, where information is presented to the learner, and it is expected that he be able to reproduce it as accurately as possible. However, memory is a skill that is also of great importance to the reading act. For example, recognizing the shapes of the different letters comprising a particular word is an act of memory. Every word also consists of letters in a particular sequence, and one has to remember what word is represented by the sequence of letters in question. Simply by changing the sequence of the letters in name, it can become mean or amen.   It is widely accepted that learning-disabled students have poor memories. "One of the most commonly described characteristics of learning-disabled students is their failure to remember important information." Although there is a large number of other "disabilities" to be found within the learning disabilities field, a reading disability — or dyslexia — remains the most commonIt is well-recognised that dyslexic students have poor memories now we understand why when internal speeches lacking memory has no prompt you see it but do not have the ability two process it internally.

Gary this makes so much sense now I know these students have not developed inner speech it explains their memory problems. Gary do you suffer with a poor memory? Yes all of my life I have had a week memory I could never remember names of people even though I re-hears them many times but when you think how important memory is in learning you begin to understand why we have these problems.

Studies have demonstrated that beginning and poor readers typically comprehend text better after reading orally rather than silently, whereas more advanced readers tend to show superior understanding after silent reading. Recently, researchers have referred to Vygotsky's sociohistorical theory when interpreting these results. The purpose of the present study was to construct in greater detail an explanatory model for these findings using Vygotskian concepts such as internalization and egocentric speech, and to assess and further develop this model with an empirical study. The reading comprehension of 73 children in grades 2, 3, and 4 was determined after they read oral and silent reading passages. In order to separate grade-level and competency-level effects, the children's teachers rated the students' reading competency, and their ratings were used as a covariate. It was expected that grade 2 and 3 children would comprehend text better after oral reading, whereas it was predicted that the grade 4 pupils would show greater understanding after silent reading. The predictions were partially supported. It was found that the grade 2 students' comprehension scores did not differ significantly between the two modes. In contrast, grade 3 and 4 students' comprehension scores were significantly higher after oral reading. Although all of the predictions were not confirmed, it is argued that the findings are consistent with a Vygotskian model of the transition from oral to silent reading. Results are discussed in terms of Vygotsky's ideas, and suggestions for Mastering the Alphabetic Principle What's the link between speed and reading in children with dyslexia? Learning to speak is a natural process, which follows a certain pattern. But, around 14-20% of pre-school children, and 5% of school-age children have problems with language – though usually these are temporary and nothing to worry about.Part of the controversy over whether people with dyslexia have general problem rapidly processing information or a problem specific to language stems from researchers' different

DOES THE RESEARCH FIT TOGETHER

You have to give it to the academics they have done their research on speech but did you hear the lack of internal speech no the unknown factor very important but unknown. It is a piece of the jigsaw puzzle what they yet have not found this piece would improve their theorys don't you think.

Gary why do you think internal speech has not had indepth research before? I honestly do not know it was talked about back in 1908 but never picked up on it, it is important for reading and writing without it you're so disadvantaged .

THINKING ABOUT INNER SPEECH

Think about this process?.. You are reading this page what are you hearing internally ?... Can you hear your voice? is it like when you're talking to someone?.. It could be something you have never thought about before?. .Lets say that you are talking to yourself internally, when did you start doing this? Can you remember? Were you taught? Did somebody say this is what you must do? Imagine this, you're reading but your internal voice switches off how difficult would reading be now?....

These are some problems that dyslexics suffer with, without the aid inner speech.

Difficulty repeating what is said to them

Difficulty comprehending written or spoken directions

Difficulty understanding or remembering what is said to them.

Difficulty understanding or remembering what they have just read.

Difficulty putting their thoughts on paper

Would they have the same difficulties if inner speech was working correctly? Try to remember if at any time your internal speech switched off? was it through being under pressure, or through anger, everyone has experienced this, but imagine this every single day no inner speech, nothing! being left disorientated, losing track of conversations, feeling out of control, how hard would things be experiencing this . Think about this lets look at your day?.. how many times are you using internal speech, take a moment and think about It? what were you doing when you are thinking about it? were you using internal speech when thinking this? I rest my case you are using it nearly all of the time.... Internal speech is a process that you use subconsciously, you don't even think about it, its automatic. It develops when you are learning to read at school the better you are at reading the stronger the internal speech unlike verbal speech " to talk out " however, verbal speech is monitored if you have a problem help is available however internal speech has never been recognised as a problem through school or every day life. In my opinion internal speech is more important than verbal speech if your internal speech is weak your verbal speech will also be weak, consequently creating confusion,complications, and problems with miss- understandings

WHY DO CHILDREN TALK TO THEMSELVES?

Whether you are a parent, teacher, or a child observer you may have noticed that many children talk to the mselves Why do children do this? Vygotsky's theories addressed Child development speaking and thinking The first stage of child development verbalised speech that helps the child to communicate with people around them . Its fasinating to watch a chid play to have a conversation with them selves you have probably scene children do this when they are playing, but why do they do this, you will often see the child playing alone having a running commentary with themselves or you can see the child organising what they are going to do they will say I need paper pencils and a pair of scissors they are not talking to anyone but themselves, this is egocentric speech that we all develop at an early stage in life we speak out before we speak in.

...

WORK ON SPEECH VYGOTSKY

Vygotsky's most important contribution concerns the inter-relationship of language development and thought. This concept, explored in Vygotsky's book Thinking and Speaking, establishes the explicit and profound connection between speech (both silent inner speech and oral language), and the development of mental concepts and cognitive awareness (<u>metacognition</u>). Inner speech is not comparable in form to external speech. External speech is the process of turning thought into words. Inner speech is the opposite, it is the conversion of speech into inward thought . When using inner speech you are reaching a higher mental functioning inner speech its connected to reason and logic, you think about the problem inwardly then come up with the answer you can debate the problem with yourself . But the Child who has not developed inner speech will not be using reason and logic in the same way yes they will have the answer but how did they get it some dys-lexics are good at mathematics they will look at the question and give you the answer but if you asked them how they got the answer they do not know something that people find strange but to me its a normal process. If I have a problem I leave it and maybe that day or the fol-lowing day the answer just comes to me, did I think about it logically was it a conscious effort NO.. the answer just came maybe from my subconscious, you find people who have dyslexia have this is common . When inner- speech is being developed the person is slowing down their thoughts they are now thinking in words,but the person who does not develop inner speech will not slow down the thought proc-ess they will be thinking too quickly and not allowing the process to take place. This will affect their understanding when communicat-ing with other people . e.g You're having a conversation with another person there is a question involved…it is important you remember the question they need an answer from you but not right away.. you have to continue listening to the lenghty conversation..plus remember-ing the question you have to answer.. you can not do it, you have to answer the question right away or you will forget what the question was because you have not developed the inner-speech where you can talk and remember questions at the same time words tend to fall out of your head because you can not see them… This can be like you are in control of conversatons however, it is not that you will find that a dyslexic will interupt during conversatons this is because if they don't say it right away they will forget what they wanted to say.. Another e.g of Inner-speech on a visit to New York friends of mine told me that when they were walking around the City, they found that people were shouting at them selves after asking why they did this the people answered because it is that noisy we can not here ourselves think we have to shout so we don't forget what we have to do or where we have to go, all this through noise imagin that all the time even when its quite you have not got a sound in your head…

EMOTIONAL TURMOIL

when internal speech is being developed it is also developing other processes reason and logic the ability to think of a problem and come up with the answer logically slowing down the way that you think thinking in the speed of speech you will find people who have not developed internal speech will be more emotional they react off emotion it reminds me of the Young Child who will not take no for an answer no reason no logic whatever you say I just want it . When I'm in this state it is addictive multiple pictures running through my mind my movements speed up my speech speeds up in fact I leave words out completely speech becomes to slow it feels clumsy and people around me seem like they're moving in slow motion to the outside world it looks like ADHD but it is not ADHD it's the brain moving at such a fantastic rate.

INNER SPEECH AND OFFENDERS

recently I interviewed a number of young offenders who had been through the Legal System they have all had learning difficulties John was in Court for stealing and driving away a vehical he had a obsession with motor vehicles I asked him why did he do it? his answer was very strange I don't know, he said I don't know why I did it… tthew was in trouble because he was caught Breaking and Entering again I asked the same question why did you do it? and once again the same answer I don't know . what did these young offenders have in common, they both came from broken backgrounds raised by their Mothers but the most interesting factor is they were both dyslexic and both showed intelligence I could say they were both above-average intelegence What was missing, it was quite clear" internal speech" internal speech had not been developed this made me think what was lacking "conscience" but what is conscience, conscience is that small voice in your mind you know what I am talking about,if you've done something wrong and that voice your mind tells you, its your choice if you carry on or not… and you can say what if I get cought?. These young males seem like they did not have the conscience that prompt you to stop you from doing it .I believe they were missing conscience conscience is developmental it is a part of internal speech without it you're totally disadvantaged why is over 50% of the prison population dyslexic and young offenders may be up to 80% have dyslexia I now believe these people never developed internal speech maybe their conscience had not developed They react to a situation emotionally no thought just sheer emotion they are not thinking about what they're doing they respond to the situation good or bad theres no thought just feelings, if this theory is correct and the biggest percentage of people who commit crime are they lacking internal speech and from this the internal conscience has not been developed, wouldn't you say this is extremely important in stopping crime today but once again people are not aware of this unknown factor. When I looked at the figures of prison, and young offenders, it did not seem right that these percentages were so great yes, we take into consideration their surroundings however the area of inner-speech needs to be acknowledged with research carried out….

WHAT IS CONSCIENCE

Conscience plays a very important role in our every day lives it lives in our Actions, our thoughts, and our feelings.It provides us with how we conduct ourselves with other people socially or privately.With our conscience it can help us with our judgment how we deal with conflict and problems before we perform our actions . Conscience is that inner voice inside our heads that warns us of danger, or wrong doings, "you will hurt that person or animal if you do that " the conscience is so important during our every day lives…You dont have oneThis can caurse major concerns for the indevidual… "not to have a conscience not to have that inner voice this is an accident waiting to happen able to construct your own thought patterns the basic facts that prompts your understanding, Education, and life skills.With recent Research it clearly showed that dyslexics have none or very little "like a whisper" had no "inner-speech" what we call conscience…. Not to make any assumptions but if we look at the prison and young offenders, what is in their head when commiting a crime From the research it is clearly stated over 50% of the prison population and young offenders suffer with dyslexia my question is why is this percentage so great surely if we go on the national averages 10% of people suffer with dyslexia so 10% of the prison population should be dyslexic not 50% we could ask our selves why is this….. Yes we must take into consideration environment, education, social skills, however the percentage is unusually high. There must be another factor something these people have in common something that clearly disadvantages them. We know that a large percentage of dyslexic people have not developed internal speech however like I said internal speech is a part of the conscience internal speech is that little voice in your mind and if you have not developed internal speech you will not have the voice that tells you what is right or wrong the lack of internal speech = lack of conscience" you can not have one without the other". Could this be the result why so many dyslexics are in prison they have not developed conscience. A screening study was undertaken which involved 50 young offenders, serving sentences of various lengths, they were all from the largest young offenders' institution in Scotland. All 50 offenders were screened for dyslexia and a number of them received a more detailed follow-up assessment. The results of the screening showed that 25 of the young offenders (50%) were some degree dyslexic. This finding has implications for professionals, particularly in respect of follow up assessment and support, and for politicians in relation to issues such as school experience, prison education and staff training. These issues are discussed here in relation to the background and results of the studyCommonly used metaphors refer to the "voice of conscience" or "voice with And a similar percentage was found in our prison populations over 50% were dyslexic. Could this really be a factor that has not been recognised in the prison population surely there must be something to explain the large percentage of people in our young offenders institute's and prisoners who are dyslexic just looking at the backgrounds and there underachieving in the education system should not be enough we have discovered a part of their development is missing could this explain why there is a need fro more research on the subject, but in my personal experience it is their lack of internal speech the lack of conscience .Concept - Inner Speech: Inner speech is the name generally used to describe the phenomenon of silent speech. It is the name given to the form of human thinking which involves (a) generating, and (b) listening back to, a stream of unspoken speech. It is holding a conversation in your own mind. It is thinking to you. Amongst the early workers with dyslexia, Huey (1908 recognised that inner speech played a major part in successfully processing textual input. The phenomenon was then a major part of Vygotsky's (1934 Key) Three-Stage Theory of Speech Development.

VYGOTSKY'S THREE-STAGE THEORY OF SPEECH DE-VELOPMENT

1st stage- Social speech (or external speech)

"In no way is this speech related to intellect or thinking."(Luria, 1992) In this stage a child uses speech to control the behavior of others. A child uses speech to express simple thoughts and emotions such as crying, laughter and shouting. An example of speech in this stage is "I want milk."

2nd stage- Egocentric Speech

This is typically the type of speech found in a three to seven year old. "It serves as a bridge between the primitive and highly public social speech of the first stage and the more sophisticated and highly private In this stage, children often talk to themselves, regardless of someone listening to them. They think out loud in an attempt to guide their own behaviour. They may speak about what they are doing.

3rd stage- Inner Speech This is the final stage of speech development.

I"inner speech". This is the type of speech used by older children and adults. This type of speech allows us to direct our thinking and behaviour. Once one has reached this final stage they are able to engage in all forms of_higher mental functions.

Gary Vygotsky he seems like an amazing man ? yes Vygotsky I could not read enough about him is work was in the 1930s he was before his time so many answers in fact my theory came from him once I realized the importance of speech development .

TESTING PEOPLE FOR INNER SPEECH

Could there be an epidemic that is unknown? has it been over-looked, could there be a large percentage of people who have not de-veloped speech correctly. Could this be the answer to the problems we have today in our schools we have problems with truancy in our schools and some students are failing we are aware of this problem but where do you start... We needed to find out how many people have this condition and does it affect learning I contacted Professor Rod Nicolson, of Sheffield University, Prof Nicolson ,and Professor Angela Fawcett is a psychologists with many years experience in learn-ing development and dyslexia, could he help? would he be open to suggestion, would he look at my theories and take them seriously.I met Professor Nicolson and Dr Angela Fawcett now herself a Professor, to discuss what I had found they showed interest they suggested creating a test that would test the " inner speech". People tested 2700 We did the research on a 2600 pupils on the inner-speech.. we asked each child to clamp the tongues between their teeth whist reading this was to stop the mouth from moving and to read in their heads... 94% out of 100% had not got the ability to do it...

They clearly had no inner-speech at all or it sounded like a whisper like someone far away..... The research will show whether 'internal speech' - the ability to process and understand words " without hav-ing to mouth them out loud" could be the missing link in develop-ing fluent reading skills.Children with dyslexia and Attention Deficit Hyperactivity Disorder are among the large numbers of people who are thought to have problems hearing words in their heads when they read silently. And this lack of an inner voice could also be contribut-ing to pupils misbehaving, with them acting out in frustration when they struggle in class.The research is being carried out by Psychologists from Sheffield University, who have linked up with Stoke-on-Trent Dyslexia Campaigner Gary Chevin to test the theory. An unnamed High School has agreed to give the questionnaires up to 1,000 of their pupils .If the results show a pattern, more trials will be carried out in other areas across the Country.Ultimately, researchers say the work could have major national implications and even influence the way children learn how to read.The Pupils will work through a series of tasks twice - once under 'normal' conditions, the other time while clamping their tongues between their teeth and lips.The two sets of data will be compared to see if there is an impact on their ability to read and interpret text when they prevent themselves mouthing or muttering the words.Mr Chevin, who lives in Sneyd Green and recently stood as a candidate in the Stoke-on-Trent mayoral election, said: "We first need to get a clearer picture of the problem. After that, we can look at developing programmes which schools could use to improve children's reading and communication skills."He is convinced people can overcome difficulties if they practise hard enough and use the right mental pointers, including step-by-step memory techniques. We will discuss this later in the book…Kathie.Mcinnes jounilist….The British dyslexia association conference 2008

INNER SPEECH AND DYSLEXIA: IS THERE A DELAY?

Angela J. Fawcett[1], Gary Chevin[2] and Roderick I. Nicolson[3]

[1] **Centre for Child Development, Swansea University**
[2] **Chevin Associates, Stoke on Trent**
[2] **Department of Psychology, University of Sheffield**

Skilled reading involves silent speech, which is scaffolded by the 'inner speech' that typically develops from 5 to 8 years, and forms the basis for thought (Vygotsky). Inner speech was considered a critical component of reading until the 1980s. We present studies indicating that inner speech increases in fluency from 6 to 10 years, and that children at risk of dyslexia typically show less developed inner speech. The process of speech internalisation is considered as an example of skill proceduralisation. Furthermore, it is likely that inner speech scaffolds many phonological skills, and, if so, the findings have important applied implications. one of the most simplest ways to check if internal speech has developed correctly was devised by Prof Nicolson, tap your finger on a table five times and get the student to count it internally see if they can do this without making a mistake do it a number of times varying how many taps you do the test , we developed must allow the person to use and manipulate inner speech, it must be something that is external, then you must go internal to use it, we came up with the number test this is taking 26 numbers that you must do… Say one out loud, and two and three internal, and carry on all the way through to 26.

THIS IS HOU IT LOOKS

1 2 3 4 5 6 7 8 9 10 11 12 13 14 15 16 17 18 19 20 21 22 23 24 25 26.

THIS IS HOW YOU DO IT

Say(1) out loud (2 3) internal, these are the numbers you will be saying out loud .

1 4 7 10 13 16 19 22 25

this test should not take more than 40 seconds to complete you must make sure the person doing it clamps their Tongue between their teeth when counting "inward" and make sure they do not move their hands or feet when doing it we also used the alphabet

First make sure the person knows the alphabet then go through the same process .

A B C D E F G H I J K L N M O P Q R S T U V W X Y

One out loud and four internally these are the answers

A F K P U Z.

These tests are getting the person to use and manipulate internal speech the person who has developed it will have no problems doing it. Each test takes 40 seconds to complete .I contacted local schools and asked if they would take part using children who had been tested for Learning Difficulties .I arranged to go in to test the students each test would take eight minutes it soon became clear a large percentage of the students could not complete the test you could see them getting confused and losing their place the inner speech what was necessary to keep them on track this was clearly not happening the inner prompt was nonexistent .

Gary did you develop these tests ? yes once I realised what was missing by talking to my wife she explained what she did and what I could not do I just came up with these tests . John... was 12 years of age he came to me late afternoon he was dyslexic I asked him if he enjoyed school he glared at me NO I hate it, I asked him why, he had come from Isolation he said I climbed on the roof and would not come down why did you do this ? I wanted them to expel me. I couldn't believe it, in 2007 a student would go to such a great lengthe to get out of school the roof was two-stories high approx 40 ft.He has just put himself in danger and what did the school do put him back in Isolation John ... could not complete the test numbers, internal speech had not developed . but when speaking to him he showed a level of maturity and intelligence . this experience brought hidden memories flooding back to me you never forget them, it left me feeling sad .Liegh... was 14 years of age he was very angry he sat with his arms folded did not smile grunted when answering could not complete the number test or complete the alphabet, his teachers said , a lost cause could liegh be heading for young offenders and may be prison, he is hiding behind a shield, uses fighting to protect himself, he has dyslexia with no internal speech develop." I wish him luck and hope he gets a lucky break"Amy.... was nine years old a pleasant child, her parents were concerned her anxiety was growing she said she hated herself and was caught knocking her head against wall, she also could not complete the numbers she could not complete the alphabet"inner speech" underdeveloped..

Margaret was 58 years old she had problems with numbers, also had problems with letters, she had worked in the Local Industry most of her life which she did not enjoy.. she felt a failure she had suffered with Depression most of her life taking Tranquillisers she said she had contemplated suicide more than once it was quite obvious she had a difficult life however, she was an Intelligent lady she had never been tested for dyslexia but she showed all the symptoms . She found it hard to follow communication at times getting frustrated and Interupting in the conversation before other person had finished speaking her inner-speech and short term memory was very weak her self-esteem was very low David… 28 years old he had problems with numbers also had problems with letters, he found out at school that he has dyslexia… he was expelled from school he got into trouble with the police on a number of occasions but joined the Army he now believes it saved him from going to prison. Now he is married, David, always day dreams and his wife often said to him what are you thinking about? David said nothing, his wife could not understand what he meant by this… it was only after we showed her the results that is inner speech was poor she began to understand. David did not think in the conventional way using words he was using pictures and working as a security guard when given the tasks he couldn't remember what to do . After explaining to David and his Wife she could not believe it she said all of our problems now make sense . Edward…. was 62 years old he also had problems with numbers also problems with letters, the test created a great deal of anxiety for him at one stage I thought he was going to cry, at the end he said he had a headache. Edward had worked in construction as a labourer he had always rejected promotion of any kind everything was done by his wife he reminded me of a child being looked after by his mother . Edwards self-esteem was very low he had suffered with anxiety nearly all of his life had taken prescription drugs .Matthew…. was a 14-year-old boy, I was asked to go visit him he was going to be expelled from his school he was creating problems in the classroom and truancy he was on his last chance.I met him on the Monday morning, I decided I was not going to lecture him I needed to find out what he was interested in. Our first meeting was very cold he did not say much after two or three meetings he started to open up and told me he had an interest in Engineering, it became clear he was dyslexic suffering with all the problems that dyslexic students have in school, but he had not been assessed this concerned me he was 14 years of age two more years left at school and he had not been assessed.I asked him Would he be interested in visiting a Local Engineering Company he jumped at the chance so I arrange for him to go and visit the Company.. We visited two weeks later he met the engineers and asked them what he needed to become an engineer he got concerned when he realised he needed qualifications he panicked at this point .

After the visit I sat down with him and drew up a plan of action of what he needed to do to reach his goal attending was a teacher who started to help him, I arranged for him to be trained on software that he could use to help him with his reading and writing, she agreed, I then made him aware of what he had to do and change his opinion on school, make him try to understand it was a start where he could reach his goal.

Instead of a negative place what only gave him grief it was to my opinion due to is dyslexic problems this had created confusion and frustration and created a negative opinion on school no one had seemed to shown him the benefits of school or taken out the time to find out what he wanted he had suffered all the through school.

He is now in his final year truanting has stopped his behaviour in class has improved and he is on target to achieve his qualifications that will allow him to go to college to become an Engineer.

Gary how did you feel working with these people ? I saw myself in all of them it was very painful at times but I needed to do the research I'm glad I did it .

Doing something about it

Sophie was a first-year law student when I met her, one-day I was watching her reading what was she doing? as she was reading to herself she was not internalising her reading her lips were moving she was whispering to herself.

I asked her could she read a paragraph to herself without moving her lips I made sure she clamped her lips tight then she tried to read she could not read anything when her lips were clamped.I explained to her she was not using internal speech she was shocked when I explained people talk to themselves internally. I tested her she had problems with numbers also letters she showed dyslexic symptoms but she had never been tested.

She had problems remembering the information she was learning her memory was weak she worked on my program for dyslexia, and over the next 12 months she made a conscious effort to internalise the information when reading and make sure she was not whispering. When meeting her 12 months later she explained her understanding and remembering had improved by 75% she had created a new habit when reading she does

not move her mouth or whisper her understanding had improved because she had made the effort to internalise information , she was reading .How many other people have this problem when reading they move their mouth and whisper be aware of people around you notice what they're doing when reading to themselves see how many of them use whispering.All of these people showed strong dyslexic symptoms they all suffered with anxiety of one degree or another, they had had very poor experiences throughout their lives it was clear inner speech was lacking and it was a factor in most of their problems they were not aware of this problem when I explained you could see relief on their faces .When you are doing these tests what are you doing you're saying 1 out loud then in your head you're saying 2 and 3 internally, there should not be much difference between what you say out loud and what you're saying internally these two modes of speaking must work together with the same clarity and strength . But the problem is when the person says 1 out loud and internally it is very weak or non existent you lose where you are and get confused and have problems completing the test, verbal speech communicates to another person internal speech communicating with oneself if your internal speech is weak or nonexistent communication with yourself is poor and this is where the problem begins a large percentage of information you must take inward to understand it and to use it reading it is external you see the words on the page and through your internal speech you take the words inward the person without inner speech will not take the words inward and their understanding will be very poor .

HOW DO I THINK

When I'm thinking about something, what am I doingISvery hard to explain it has taken me a number of years to become aware of it it, starts with pictures running through my mind at a phenomenal speed we could say it is so fast it becomes outside of your knowing I have now developed the ability to slow the pictures down and see them more clearly but the problem is I do not see each stage growing I just see the end picture this becomes a problem when trying to describe a situation that needs detail I have no detail in my thoughts. This answers the question about the young dyslexic who is good at mathematics he sees the problem and then sees the answer on the picture if you ask him how did you get the answer he would not know because there is no detail just the answer . He did not develop inner speech he did not develop Analytical Reason and Logic he did not think internally about the problem That's how it felt like a secret no one will tell you about the condition, looking at Dyslexia what did I find dyslexic people are, they are profound picture thinkers, their number one mode of thinking is pictures, they think too quickly they have not slowed their thought processes down by using internal speech and thinking in the speed of speech .When you are developing inner speech you are changing the pictures to words think about speaking it follows a structure and speed when inner speech is developed you now think in this speed 10.000 Pictures a Minute compared to 250 words per minute to the average reader. When you're using literacy you are following a structure it is linear, the problem is, it is developmental you must use this process but for the person who has not mastered literacy they will not have developed linear it goes hand-in-hand. Taking the information inward how do you do this process? .When you use inner-speech you see the information and take it inward with inner speech the inability to use inner- speech will stop the processing of the information.

THE SECRET WITHIN

VISUALLY DEAF AUDITORY BLIND

That's how it felt like a secret no one will tell you about the condition, looking at Dyslexia what did I find dyslexic people are, they are profound picture thinkers, their number one mode of thinking is pictures, they think too quickly they have not slowed their thought processes down by using internal speech and thinking in the speed of speech .When you are developing inner speech you are changing the pictures to words think about speaking it follows a structure and speed when inner speech is developed you now think in this speed 10.000 Pictures a Minute compared to 250 words per minute to the average reader. When you're using literacy you are following a structure it is linear, the problem is, it is developmental you must use this process but for the person who has not mastered literacy they will not have developed linear it goes hand-in-hand. Taking the information inward how do you do this process? . When you use inner-speech you see the information and take it inward with inner speech the inability to use inner- speech will stop the processing of the information. let's look at it? I see the word clearly **but can not hear it internally..** I see it but do not hear it I call this **VISUALLY DEAF...** just think about this process when you look at any written information automatically you are processing it without thinking its like a running commentary through your mind how would it feel if the running commentary switched off, you would now be **VISUALLY DEAF.. I can see it but can not hear it** . Another challenge for the dyslexic is what do you do when your spelling? people internalise the word they see it in their mind it is a prompt that helps you remember spelling, but the dyslexic cannot do this they find it virtually impossible to visualise words if you're listening to some one saying a word then ask you to spell the word.. now you have heard the word you can spell the word internally, however the dyslexic does not, I call this **AUDITORY BLIND.... I hear it but can not see it** So what is dyslexia? **VISUALLY DEAF AUDITORY BLIND** thinking too quickly and not using linear thought this is what I face on a day-to-day basis, I cannot hear the information internally I do not see the information internally my mind is working to quickly and I am not following a step-by-step process all of my problems originate from these symptoms but all of these symptoms are developmental you have to develop them nobody tells you to develop them they are left to develop on their own. The person who is not dyslexic will be using internal speech they will have the ability to visualise words

Gary visually death auditory blind how did you come up with this ? it was one of them things it just came to me no thought I just saw it .internally they will be thinking in the speed of speech and will be using linear thought. If you could not use these processes you would also be dyslexic with all of the dyslexic problems Inner speech is being developed probably by the age of 8 also the child is using spoken thought then it goes inward to become internal speech and over the next few years it is being developed to the point where it becomes automatic you don't even think about it you use it for reading processing analysing and it is connected to memory .When using it you are thinking in words slowing your thoughts to the speed of speech this process is developed subconsciously . The ability to see words….. the dyslexic has not develop this process they do not see words internally, the person who has developed this will have the ability to see the words they are spelling and by looking at the word they will know if the word is spelt correctly.

PROBLEMS WITH INNER SPEECH

the problem of the person who has not developed inner speech it will affect their ability to read effectively their processing and analysing skills will be impaired their understanding of the spoken language will be a problem they will be thinking too quickly they have not slowed their thought processes down they are not thinking in speech they are still thinking in visual image and this is an unknown condition that could affect millions of people throughout the world . People who suffer with this condition will have problems with pronunciation of words I am not sure but I believe the President of the United States of America George W Bush he often says the wrong words in the wrong order you see him delivering a speech then losing his place he is not following internal speech he cannot rehearse his speech internally Richard Branson, an entrepreneur and a billionaire you see him often losing his way when speaking Robbie Williams, he cannot keep anything inward everything comes out without thought, the young child at school who is told off for shouting out in the classroom he hears what you say and reacts to it without thought . If I look back throughout my life it's there I reacted without thought it is a problem maybe what the young offender has you can do something without thinking could this be why they get into trouble? it isn't only when you're learning it affects you it effects you throughout your life. You must understand all of these problems are developmental you can develop them "inner speech" is developmental it is speech, and speech is tought you must know what to do and how to do it you must slow down the way you are thinking and learn to think in linear one step at a time but how do you do this . you must understand we have a strong tendency to think in pictures picture thinking is natural we do it, from a very early age . so to create

Gary Chevin

internal speech we will use pictures, pictures that give you sounds and a pictorial prompt which you can follow .

LEARNING WITHOUT INNER SPEECH THINKING IN 3 PICTURES

we must understand the problems the person faces who has not developed internal speech they are thinking too quickly they have not slowed the thought processes down by thinking with speech their thoughts are pictorial the first thing you must do is slowdown your thoughts and think in linear you need to think step-by-step .

we are going to copy the process used when reading we must take it from external then go internal getting the mind to manipulate the information . We are going to use numbers .

1 2 3 4 5 6 7 8 9 10 11 12 13 14 15 16 17
18 19 20 21 22 23 24 25 26

number 1 I want you to imagine a candle the candle is long and thin it looks like number **1** when you see **1** think od candle

1 Candles

number 2… I want you to imagine twins when you think of **2** think of twins .

2 Twins…..

number 3… I want you to imagine a **3** leg stool when you think of **3** you see the **3** leg stool .

3 Stool….

number 4… I want you to imagine a car a car has **4** wheels so when you see the number **4** you think of car .

4 Car….

60

number 5... I want you to imagine your hand your hand has **5** fingers when you see, the number **5** you think of hand .

5 Hand....

number 6.... **6** sounds like bricks when you see the number **6** think of bricks

6 Bri

number 7... I want you to imagine a lucky charm when you think of **7** you think of lucky charm

7 Charm....

number 8.... when you see **8** it sounds like plate so if you see **8** you think of plate .

8 Plate....

number 9.... I want you to imagine a black cat why a cat? a cat has **9** lives when you see **9** you think of cat .

9 Cat....

number 10.... I want you to imagine number **10** Downing Street it's where the Prime Minister lives when you see **10** you think of the door

10 Door....

let's go through the numbers number **1** candle. number **2** twins. number **3** stool. number **4** car. number **5** hand. number **6** bricks. number **7** charm. number **8** plate. number **9** ca.t number **10** door .

number 11.... I want you to imagine a foot ball team there are **11** players in a football team when you see **11** you think of football .

11 Football

number 12.... I want you to imagine **12** eggs there are **12** eggs to the dozen when you see **12** you think of eggs

12 Eggs..

number 13... I want you to imagine a witch the witch flies on Friday the**13tth**   when you see **13** you think of witch .

13 Witch

number 14... I want you to imagine gold **14** ^ gold when you see **14** you think of gold .

14 Gold

number 15... I want you to imagine coffee beans **15** and bean sound the same when you see **15** you think of bean.

15 Bean

number 16... I want you to imagine sweet **16** when you see **16** you think of sweet **16**

16 Sweet.

number 17... I want you to imagine Ward **17** where you visit your friend "hospital" when you see **17** you think of Ward **17**

17 Ward.

number 18... I want you to imagine a pint of beer you can drink beer when you're **18** when you see **18** you think of beer .

18 Beer.

number 19.... I want you to imagine the clubhouse on a golf course whole number **19** is the clubhouse .

19 Club House.

number 20... I want you to imagine **20** sticks tied together when you see **20** you think of sticks .

20 sticks.

number 21... I want you to imagine a birthday cake when you're **21** it's a big birthday so if you see **21** you think of cake .

21 Cake.

number 22… I want you to imagine carrot there are **22** carat gold forget the gold and think of carrot when you see **22** you think of carrot .

22 Carrot.

number 23… I want you to imagine a flee when you see **23** it sounds like flee .

23 Flee.

number 24… I want you to imagine Christmas Eve the night before Christmas this night is where most people cook their turkey when you see **24** think of Turkey.

24 Turkey.

number 25… I want you to imagine a Christmas tree people have a Christmas tree at Christmas when you see **25** you think of tree .

25 Tree. number 26… the day after Christmas is called Boxing Day when you see , **26** you think of box .

26 Box.

You now have learnt 26 new pictures these pictures relate to numbers try this what is the picture for number **4** what is the picture for number **10** what is the picture for number **21** what is the picture of number **5** you can play with this like it is a game get to know all the pictures and put them with the numbers .the answer **CAR, DOOR, CAKE, HAND,** keep on going through them untill you know them without thinking. We are now going to use these to emulate the process of thinking internally, slowing the student down and thinking in linear. Once you have learnt these pictures "try this" make sure there are two or three people in the room the first person says candle the second person says twins carry on around the room untill you get to 26 try to keep it in order then try to go backwards from 26 to 1 "keep it fun"

I want you to remember these numbers .

1 3 9 4 10 1 5 7 3 1

How do you remember these numbers first change the numbers into the pictures **Witch, cat, car, bean, lucky-charm, stool, candle.** this is how you do it . The **witch** and the **cat** landed on a **car** opened the door and took a **bean** that looked like a **lucky-charm** they sat on a **stool** and lit a **candle.**Learn this story who was with the witch? what did they land on? what did the bean look like? what did they light? go through the story 2 or 3 times then get some one to ask you questions on it . You now know the story we are now going to change the pictures to the numbers **witch 13, cat 9, car 4, door 10, bean 15, charm 7, stool 3, candle 1,** and this is how it looks **1 3 9 4 1 0 15 7 3 1** get some one to ask you questions on the numbers e.g. what comes after **10** all you have to do is go through the story in your mind remember what **10** is its **door,** whats the next picture its **bean 15.** . keep practicing untill you know the story with pictures and numbers.you are slowing yourself down to the speed of speech seeing each individual piece you are now thinking in linear processing and analysing the information internally. We are now going to add to our pictures what is **1** **"candle"** the candle was pushed into an apple, now what is **2 "twins"** the twins are playing with the ball. What is **3 "stool"** a cat is sitting on the **"stool"** what is **4 "car"** the dog has jumped on a **"car"** what is **5 "hand"** in your hand you are holding a egg

let's look at them again

1 candle Apple

2 twins ball

3 stool cat

4 car dog

5 hand egg

Now make sure you have learnt these first five before carrying on. What are the pictures for **2** its **twins** they are playing with a ball, when remembering these try to see them in your mind like a cartoon see the **twins** playing with a ball that is as big as a car. Now what is the picture for **candle** its **1** see in your mind a large apple then stick the apple into the candle. Now what is the picture for **6** its **bricks** imagin your making a fish tank out of **bricks** think its **fish tank.** Now what is the picture for **7** its **lucky-charm** the lucky charm is around the **goats neck** lucky charm its **goats neck..** Now what is the picture for **8** its **plate** the plate turns into a **hat** plate its **hat.** Now what is the picture for **9** its **cat** the cat lives in a **Igloo** cat **Igloo.** Now what is the picture for **10** its **door** the Prime Minister came through the **door** and the **jelly** was thrown at him **door jelly** let's look at these five

6 bricks fish

7 charm goat

8 plate hat

9 cat igloo

10 door jelly.

Again go through these five making sure you know both pictures. What are the pictures for **8** its **plate** draw a picture of a **plate** turning into a **hat** make it funny make it silly .it helps if you draw pictures of both pictures together what is the picture for **11 football** a **kite** is tied to the **football** its **kite football.** What is the picture for **12 eggs** the eggs are covered by **leaves** its **eggs leaves.** What is the picture for **13** its **witch** the **witch** is flying past the **moon** its **witch moon.** what is the picture for **14** its **gold** the gold is in a **nest** its **gold nest.** What is the picture for **15** its **bean** the bean turns into a **orange bean** its **orange.** let's look at these five

11 football kite

12 eggs leaves

13 which moon

14 gold nest

15 bean orange

What is the picture for **16** its **sweets** the **penguin** is eating **sweets** its **sweets penguin.** What is the picture for **17** its   **ward** the **queen** visits the **ward** its **ward queen.**   What is the picture for **18** its **beer** a **ring** falls into the **beer** its **beer ring.** What is the picture for **19** **clubhouse** the **sun** was shining on the **clubhouse** its **sun clubhouse.** What is the picture for sticks **20** its **sticks** they fell out of the **tree.** let's look at these five

16 sweets Penguin

17 ward queen

18 beer ring

19 clubhouse sun

20 sticks tree

What is the picture for **21** its **cake** the **cake** was in the shape of an **umbrella** its **cake umbrella.** What is the picture for **22** its **carrots** the **carrot** was in a **vase** its **carrots vase.** What is the picture for **23** its **flee** the **flee** was on a **whale** its **flee whale.** What is the picture for **24** its **turkey** the **turkey** went for a **x-ray** its **turkey x-ray.** What is the picture for **25** its **christmas tree** the **christmas tree** turned **yellow** its **christmas tree yellow.** What is the picture for **26 box** in the **box** there was a **zebra** its **box zebra.** let's look at these five

21 cake Umbrella

22 carrots vars

23 flee whail

24 Turkey x-ray

25 Christmas tree yellow

26 box zebra

let's go through them all

    1 candle apple **2** twins bal.l **3** stool cat. **4** car dog. **5** hand egg. **6** bricks fish. **7** charm goat. **8** plate hat. **9** cat igloo. **10** door jelly. **11** football kite. **12** eggs leaves. **13** which moon. **14** gold nest. **15** bean orange. **16** sweets Penguin. **17** ward queen. **18** beer ring. **19** clubhouse sun. **20** sticks tree. **21** cake Umbrella. **22** carrots vars. **23** flee whail. **24** Turkey x-ray. **25** Christmas tree yellow. **26** box zebra. It helps to draw them it doesn't have to be brilliant just a simple drawing of both pictures. Don't continue untill you know all **26** pictures and the new **26** pictures. Its important its done this way. Listen to the story. A **penguin** in a **hat** lived in a **igloo** covered in **leaves** he liked to eat **oranges** under the **sun** he eats **oranges** and the **penguin** in the **hat** turned **yellow...** Learn the story ask questions about it, how many **oranges** did the **penguin** eat? Where did he live? what did he have on his head? what colour did he turn? now draw it. We are thinking more slowly following a sequence what is in order we are internalising the information but what did we learn? **penguin, hat, igloo, leaves, oranges, sun, oranges, penguin, hat, yellow..** We are now going to turn the picture into a letter Penguin **p** hat **h** igloo **i** leaves **L** orange **o** sun **s** orange **o** Penguin **p** hat **h** yellow **y** put them all together you have just learnt how to spell **PHILOSOPHY** you are now learning to think in words you can see the word **philosophy** now you have gone from just pictures and now you can change the pictures into letters that make up the word. Now find a word really difficult make up the story learn it then change the pictures to the letters. This method is trying to emulate what people do when reading in their heads. You must be persistent and consistent and have fun when doing it, let me ask you a question what is the 10th letter of the alphabet? don't panic you know it step **1** **10 door, step 2** the prime minister, what happens to him he gets a **jelly** throne at him step **3** the answer is **j** for **jelly.** the **10**[th] letter of the alphabet is **J.** Try another one. Try another…. 20th letter step **1 20** gives you **sticks** step **2** they fell out of a **tree** step **3** answer is **20** sticks **tree** the 20th letter of the alphabet is **t.** Get some one to write down a number and then you give the answer. What is this method doing? its slowing down the person getting them to think in linear following a structure and seeing the information internally we're trying to create the process of internal speech .I want you to go through these pictures in your mind **Apple, Ball, Cat, Dog, Egg, Fish, Goat, Hat, Igllo, Jelly, Kite, Leaves, Moon, Nest, Orange, Penguin, Queen, Ring, Sun, Tree, Umbrella, Vase, Whale X-ray, Yellow, Zebra..** go through these pictures keep them in order see them internally .Once you can do this easily I want you now to try to create the sound to each picture. **Apple** gives you **a** now keep on practising till you can **hear** the **sound internally.** It might sound like a whisper but if you keep on trying you will get a more **clear sound..** keep it fun. you now know the alphabet, you now know the position, and the structure. Once you have learnt the alphabet try to do the alphabet backwards, don't panic you know it start with the pictures **26 box** what was in the box **zebra z** next picture **25** what is the picture **tree** turning **yellow y** take your time and see each picture . Internal speech is perfected when the students take reading internally but the problem for the dyslexic students they never master reading so internal speech is never mastered we have to try to emulate the processes used when the student is mastering inner speech. Since I have been using this technique my inner speech has improved I now use a whisper I used to have nothing no sound at all what are the benefits. Communication with other people is now easier I feel like my world has slowed down allowing me to understand more of the information around me but I understand I am still developing it it may take a number of years to get to the same degree as spoken language but you can develop it .

Gary you were emulating reading ? yes I had studied what people do when reading and tried to emulate the same pattern I knew we had to slow down the way we think and get us to think in linear .**Gary** this method allowed you to learn how to spell ? yes but even more than that it allowed me to remember the spelling and how the spelling was made up .

THE DEFECT

When carrying out this research we discovered other defects in inner speech something that shocked me. It was my wife when reading she used inner speech it was perfect the same strength and clarity as verbal speech but when she was using mathematics something happened she has problems with mathematics she does not understand them when watching her she emulates a dyslexic person first confusion takes over her she cannot internalise the information she verbalises the information outward, when asking her what is happening she cannot see the information internally her inner speech switches off.Could confusion destroy inner speech? When the person gets confused does inner speech turnoff my wife has perfect inner speech untill she uses mathematics this creates confusion and inner speech is turned off could that be one of the answers why inner speech does not develop. we know that fear affects internal speech have you ever been in a situation where you were frightened e.g you may be delivering a presentation you're Scared and nervous and you lose what you're going to say your inner speech switched off and you lost your place. But there was another problem my wife faced when she was reading to herself internally she suffered with an internal stutter she would be reading normal then get stuck on a word she can read it but she cannot say it, it kept on repeating and repeating in her mind this destroys the ability to read on whatever she does she cannot move forward she is now disadvantaged. The problem is if she is in a examination and the internal stuttering starts she cannot go forward, whatever she tries to do she is stuck how common is this. When I was working in the primary schools I went into three classrooms and asked if anyone suffers with the internal stutter over 50% of the students recognised it and had experienced it.I met a 16-year-old girl who had just left school she showed dyslexic symptoms she told me she experiences the internal stutter and how it destroyed her in the examinations, she told me about an examination she took at the beginning of the examination the stutter started and she could not move forward as hard as she tried she could not move onwards she did not finish the examination and she failed. The internal stutter is just as unknown as the lack of internal speech it is quite obvious these speech problem affect the students in a dramatic way but they are unknown. Academics are not aware of them they cripple and destroy the students ability to achieve they don't only affect students who have special needs it may affect up to 50% of the students and school pupils today. This problem needs to be addressed.We know that verbalise speech can have problems when developing could this also affect internal speech they are both to do with speech and I would imagine they both could develop incorrectly however we know when some one has a problem with verbal speech there are speech therapists to help but what if internal speech is affected what help could you get no one who is aware of this condition something that concerns me.Over the last nine years I have been proactive in the world of dyslexia I was the vice-chairman of the local Dyslexia Association working very close with the British Dyslexia Association, also Dyslexia Action I travelled all over the UK working on problems with Dyslexia.

Gary you've explained about inner speech but inner starter what is this ? The research was so new and different things just appeared I do not suffer with the inner stutter you must have a degree of inner speech to suffer with this it needs more research .

In 1999 I worked with my Local MP the LEA and Colleges and Business to raise funds for the Dyslexia Community not forgetting Dyslexic Adults we raised £1 million for a Dyslexia Centre.After working for two years on this project I created two positions one with the LEA and one with the Local College the position with the college was what I had been doing for 2 yrs now you must remember that this new post was developed along side the head of department for learning stratagies together we did the job discription and what was needed for this particular position. I had been working with this pogram for 2 yrs developing it and constructing it, you would think that the best person for this post would be the one who created it. The postion was advertised in the local newspaper and Jobcener Plus.. of cause I had to go through all the proper chanals just like the other canidates did, when my interveiw came they asked me about my knowledge in this area and funding I had raised they did not know that I had developed it as things had to be on each indevidual merit. When the letter came saying unsuccessful I could not believe it I got in touch with head of department who I had been working with for the passed 2yrs and told her of the result of me not attcheiving this post she telephoned me later that day to inform me that   they had put on a qualification level

4 on the program she apologised in saying Gary you have no qualifications and it was out of her hands. I was devistated the position went to an ex fireman who had no qualifications in this area and within 16 months of his postion it ran out funding my program which was so successful was put into the hands of inexperianced staff and once again I felt like I had failed not through what I was capable of I created the program it goes to show that in Brittain it is qualification led and not ability led forget what you know forget what you can do forget what you have developed if you have no qualifications you don't stand a chance, to give the position to an ex-fireman who has know knowledge in dyslexia or fund raising is very poor judgment on the staff who did the interveiws. It was my work and skill that they were using and within 16 months he failed.

Gary how did this affect you ? I could not believe it I had done all the work I had been on all the meetings my ideas this and at the end of the day it meant nothing because Gary had not got any qualifications surely this is wrong .

A head teacher in Cheshire heard about what I was doing and approached me she had two dyslexic sons I arranged to go and visit her and started to work with her youngest son after six weeks his spelling improved his mathematics improved his memory also improved he was having private lessons for mathematics one-day he was explaining to his tutor how he could see mathematics his tutor was amazed he was talking about pictures what turned into numbers .The head teacher was amazed with his progress and asked if I would be willing to do some research, I agreed she arranged for me to go into three primary schools and three secondary schools to carry out research

MY FIRST DAY BACK IN SCHOOL

It was on Monday morning late in August I arrived at the school at 8:30 a.m. it was 30 years since Gary had been to school but this time I was the teacher one of the teachers had taken me to a small room at the end of the corridor I sat down and waited for seven young pupils ti arrive into the classroom there was 6 boys and 1 girl they all looked nervous not knowing Gary was more nervous than them I had decided

I must make them feel relaxed I remembered my school days and how I hated special lessons I started by saying my name is Gary if you want me you must call me Gary the look on their faces they were shocked they always had to call the teachers Miss and Sir but I wanted them to feel relaxed I was not going to lecture to them I wanted them to take part in fact I wanted them to beome the teachers .One of the most important thing is to build their confidence I knew their confidence was low I wanted them to succeed from the very beginning lose the feeling of failure and kill their self limiting believes we started… I got them to remember 26 pictures in the correct order they didn't realise they were learning they thought it was a game One of them took over and became the teacher and I became a student we played a guessing game at the end of the lesson there was a different look on their faces I felt like I had got through they were 14 years of age school had not been a pleasant experience .The second lesson they came in smiling they wanted to take part we learnt another 26 pictures they still did not know what they were learning I gave them a combination of pictures to remember they now could do it easily these were the pictures Lucky charm gold cake twins and a plate a stool and a hand a car and twins a car and a cat a hand and a brick a brick and a stool a lucky charm and an orange two Lucky charms a plate and a car then I asked them to change the pictures to numbers .Lucky charm **7** gold **14** cake **21** twins **2** and a plate **8** put them together **28** a stool **3** and a hand **5** put them together **35** a car **4** twins **2** put them together **42**.. A car **4** a cat **9** put them together **49** A hand **5** bricks **6** put them together **56** Brick **6** a stool **3** put them together **63** A lucky charm **7** orange **0** put them together **70** Two Lucky charms 77 a plate **8** and a car **4** put them together **84** what had they learned .7 **14 21 28 35 42 49 56 63 70 77 84**..

they had learnt their seven times tables without even knowing it it was done so softly they weren't even aware of it it happened naturally some people would say what a long drawnout way to learn their tables but it wasn't they learnt in a way which they would not forget they were relaxed and they enjoyed it it was more like a game not a boring lesson I just believed if I was learning something and it was boring I wouldn't learn it we need it to be enjoyable to learn effectivelWe then got to know the building blocks of words letters you need to know then to work with them . One of the most amazing things I saw in school seven dyslexic students run into the library to find the biggest word and learn how to spell it they chose their own word what was it AN-THROPOMORPIC… that was the word they chose they learnt how to spell this word in five minutes they could tell you the makeup of the word they could even spell it backwards "Amaging don't you think"… there was a transformation of the seven students their self belief grew they had done things what they couldn't do before why do so many of our students fail today I believe its confusion and sheer boredom if their lessons were made more enjoyable and fun maybe they would learn more the main focus of my lessons keep it fun and make sure they enjoy it and let them take control of their own learning . What does anthropomorphic look like internally you must be able to see it to understand it, it starts like this…Step **1** There was an apple in a nest that was in a tree. step **2** in the hat there was a ring plus an orange. step **3** a penguin eating an orange under the moon. step **4** The orange fell on a ring. step **5** a penguin in a hat lived in a igool with a cat step **6** you learn the story and learn the word you understand the makeup . Draw the story out then get some one to test you.….One thing was very clear I would say , all of the students I worked with had problems with inner speech .I worked with a student he had autism/dyslexia when I met him it was hard to get his attention is mind was everywhere I knew I had to get his attention to help him, I started him with the same pictures and I got him to draw them i could hold his attention for 15 minutes then I let him leave, we did another 15 minutes this was the only way I could get his attention with every 15 minute we had intervals. After four sessions I was now getting to 25 minutes then taking a break he was learning quickly I finally got to 30 minutes I did not want to increase any more than 30 minutes.We took a break after working 30 minutes, we would then take a 10 minute break. His father told me his attention grew at home and would I meet his teacher I gladly accepted she told me he had improved tremendously and could I show her what we had been doing I did so in fact I had a full day in her school delivering the programme to her team .but her team had problems they were nearly all verbal thinkers they had to change to pictorial to learn the programme it was strange it was like looking at students who had problems with literacy . They found it difficult to do I was teaching a pictorial alphabet that changed to letters. The students found it easy to do because they were pictorial thinkers it was more natural to them.After seven months I had completed the primary School and secondary schools the results we received were very favorable. Over the next 18 months Gary you have gone through so much with your dyslexia you have told me about what you went through but you must feel pleased with your work and how successful your work was in the school's.Yes I still go through the feelings that I had before however I can manage them better now you must understand my program is there to help and assist dyslexic's. The school's and colleges did work, however, I felt I had to take it to a different level you know to people who wont come across my work if they are not in the same field as the school's or colleges.So what did you do next to make it more available?..We turned my programme into books it was dispatched to 130 schools around the UK I was prepared to train however teachers say they know whats best training was included with training teachers so how successful it was it I don't know the parents were disapointed because they knew it was perfect for their dyslexic child I had excellent feedback from them.I remember one student in the primary School he was about nine years of age very quiet he just smiled at you he had major problems with literacy and mathematics whatever they did with him it never seemed to work his defence was say nothing just smile but it was clear to me he was suffering with mass confusion he had been confused for many years. How could I help?.. First I must help him to relax I used breathing techniques before i started then get him to take control of his own learning, help him to build his confidence and not to focus on reading, writing, and spelling, he knew he could not do these things. After severn weeks of working with him there was a dramatic change. When I had finished his mother said he now enjoys school and wants to learn. One thing I do regret not being more involved into helping schools to truly understanding the benefits of these programmes not just helping the student to read, right, spel,l and do mathematics, but to help the student to really enjoy the learning process .

Gary it seems like you enjoyed your time at school ? yes it is an amazing feeling to work with children who believed they were useless helping them to build their self-confidence and achievement was wonderful in fact it was one of the most best times of my life .

WHAT IS THOUGHT?

Are we asking the right question when we say what is thought should we be asking what develops thought, since the ancient Greeks this question has been asked so let's look at what develops developmental thought .

DO ANIMALS THINK?

A Question that I asked myself I suppose the answer would be yes they must think but we must define what we mean by thought, every year thousands of cats and dogs get killed on the roads animals react to situations when they are out on the streets they will run in front of a moving vehicle they have no developmental thought this is their problem they cannot analyse a situation they just react.Before speech developed a Child reacts in exactly the same way if the Child was in the street the Child would run in front of moving vehicles no developmental thought just reaction it is only when the Child develops speech and understanding to a degree of mastery that developmental thought will grow

THE BEGINNING

The Child is now at the age where he/she is learning how to speak, the seeds of thought are speech its developmental we are taught how to do it by our parents and carers this stage is a very important one it is were thought begins the child is learning how to sound out words and put words to objects stringing words together to make sentences very basic but the beginning of communication skills start here as the child practices speech it becomes more   fluent. At this stage could we say the child is using developmental thought that incorporates analytical reason and logic skills the answer is no the child can communicate and put words to objects but at this time developmental thought is not yet developed .

HOW DOES THOUGHT DEVELOP?

Before we look at developmental thought we should be aware of certain aspects in life we have principles and practices we tend to lean towards man's practices but the only problem with man's practice is when they go wrong we are left with a feeling of uselessness if you look round the world you can see man's practices in progress how men build houses if we look at China the houses are different the beliefs are different the language is different than it is England but nature's principles are nearly always the same. If you build a fire in England and a fire in China they will both burn with the same intensity natures principles that comes natural to us we should always be aware of this with everything we do in life.Most children when they are developing are following natures principles each stage is natural to them they laugh they sit up and then the most important aspect of nature's principal is "walking" but at this stage developmental thought is not yet developed how does it develop and what is the major influence of it? Well you have to ask yourself   when the child begins to speak developmental thought is being laid down the first stage at this point could we say the child has developmental thought they can communicate with their parents in a certain way they can play with their friends but they have not yet developed developmental thought. We must be aware of how the child is thinking the child is thinking in a natural way a principle of nature we all start out with pictorial thought we learn , and remember through pictures we know the face of our mother and father through the picture in our mind this way of thinking is natural we learn quickly we have developed the first part of thought using a pictorial thought process we could go through life okay using this way of thinking but it must change to move to the second part of developmental thought. Off we go to school and it all changes the way that we think must change to move forward the teacher says cat in our mind we see the clear precise picture of the cat but she writes on the board three letters and says cat this creates confusion from nature's principles to man's practices we must change the picture to a word some people find it easy and others virtually impossible to do. The person who finds it easy to change the picture to a word will start to develop the second part of developmental thought when they changed pictures to words something happened they had the ability to see the words, they now see the word inward once you do this you have developed inner speech as inner speech is being developed it is developing other aspects of thought analytical reason and logic skills are being developed linear thought is being developed when completed developmental thought will be in place allowing the person to learn in the conventional way and that is a major influence of thought and speech .The person who could not change the picture to a word will now be disadvantaged they won't take speech inwardly they will not develop analytical reason and logic skills they will not develop linear thought this will affect concentration, attention, and memory, and so many other aspects that will have a effect on communication skills learning will be virtually impossible at times the teacher will be thinking in a different way than the student to think will be virtually impossible at times if the pictures are not there they will not understand this will cause confusion, and frustration, and the downward spiral will begin . How is thought developed developmental thought needs speech without speech it is poor so on this understanding speech is the main influence to developmental thought, speech comes in three parts the first part verbalised speech which is taught to us by our parents and carers this is a very important part, research has been carried out in primary school children they found out the children who had not developed speech correctly would suffer in learning. Verbal speech must be developed correctly.The second part of speech egocentric speech this is when the Child speaks out their own thoughts extremely important to develop this skill this is a precursor to internal speech this internal speech it is just as important as verbalise speech when speech goes inward developmental thought is complete without this process the individual persons thought will be weak .If you find it hard to believe try to read internally without using inner speech think about "thought" are you using speech when "thinking" think about your day how many times do you talk to yourself inwardly throughout the day.Over the past five years I have researched this area it became apparent a large percentage of dyslexic people had not developed inner speech from my own experiences this was clear analysing what was happening when inner speech was not there I discovered the lack of analytical reason and logic skills linear thought was poor and memory was weak also the inability to visualize words internally. When some one develops inner speech they are slowing their thought processes down my own thought processes followed a stream of images the problem with this they were moving too quickly at times this created hyperactivity my movements and speech became erratic communication was poor and following verbal instructions was hard.Another element I discovered through the research we carried out was the internal stutter, this was totally unknown this condition could affect up to 40% of the population an unknown epidemic the people who suffered with this did not have to have learning difficulties however it could slow them down.The one area which was the most interesting was the underdeveloped developmental thought it was clear this will affect people in a dramatic way now we know how it is developed however how do we monitor the development of inner speech.This research is not complete I'm very interested to see what we will find in the future. Verbalised speech to communicate with other people Internal speech to communicate with oneself both important in communication skills if either one is poor the long-term problems will be detrimental to the person we must put a bigger emphasis on speech development this will alleviate a large percentage of problems that children experience at school. The problems what are created when inner speech is not developed can be quite intense the lack of inner speech and the lack of developmental thought will go hand-in-hand and also the lack of analytical reason and logic skills will be apparent The person who has not developed inner speech will react in a different way than some one who has developed inner speech. If a question was asked to person who has not developed inner speech their answer would be purly on feelings they would have no thought they could not analys the question to give you the answer. When you have no analytical reason or logic you tend to react on feelings, as you look at the person reacting on feelings the similarity to a Child will be very clear their reaction will emulate a child asking for something as you say no they will get more intense not accepting no the person who does not develop inner speech developmental thought will take this response all through their lives their communication skills will be very poor when in this state it will be hard to reason with them their emotions will be out-of-control tempers will explode they are reacting to your answer emotionally no thought no analyzing just sheer emotion what can create major problems .

Gary do you really believe there is aspects of thought what have not been developed ? Yes wants you understand about inner speech and how it affects the person when it has not been developed you can just see it in a person who has not developed it .

One thing that concerns me with some of the students is I have met their future in the employment market. with the verbal and written communication, linguistic difficulties they are not easy to cope with. Reading and learning go hand in hand. One must learn to read in order to be able to read to learn. A child who is a poor reader will usually also be a poor learner. Literacy is also the key to employment. Dyslexia can jeopardize a child's entire future. When your able-bodied finding employment is easy I was a builder for 24 years finding work was easy but after my accident things changed I applied for hundreds of positions and wasn't successful did I have the experience yes I had worked in schools and outside of schools with people who have dyslexia I had carried out research and worked with some of the experts in the UK you would think it would be easy but it wasn't you see Gary did not have qualifications and all the good positions needed qualifications this is when I truly understood the difficulties dyslexic people have finding employment. Recently Dyslexia Action joined With Remploy they help disabled people to find employment they acknowledge that the dyslexic community have difficulties in finding employment.I am a firm believer in education and qualifications but what happens when the student cannot take part in conventional education they go all the way through their schooling and achieve nothing they leave school with no qualifications in many cases their future is blighted .Our society today is academic based you are judged on what academic qualifications, you have, what happened to ability why should the person who has no qualifications become blocked in the employment opportunities surely we should take into consideration ability led some of our finest entrepreneurs have no qualifications they left school with nothing but had the ability to do it Richard Branson, Alan sugar, people who have no qualifications but vision and ability they certainly have.This should be taken into consideration on the applications for employment what have you done what have you achieved outside off qualifications I believe this country is missing a large percentage of untapped potential. When we think of dyslexic people what are the benefits, the benefits are to think out of the box, creative imaginations, visual, why aren't these talents used I believe the business community are not aware of this they have not been educated about the value of dyslexia. What a waste. A large percentage of dyslexic adults are unemployed due to their lack of qualifications and literacy skills and then you have got those who are in employment and refuse promotion due to paper work and book work, which maybe involved the thought of this makes them physically ill and they are ashamed of their disability and do not want their employer knowing they can not read or not read very well or their righting is poor and spelling is bad.

Gary I did not know that Dyslexia was a disability. It will be interesting to know whatrights people have. Do people know that it is classed as a disability nine out of 10 people who are dyslexic have no understanding at all that dyslexia is a disability and that is wrong there is law what protects them .

DYSLEXIA AND DISABILITY

It is well documented that there is a higher incidence of dyslexia within the prison and probation populations, those excluded from school and the long term unemployed compared to the population as a whole. The Dyslexia Institute conservatively estimates, based on the population norm for the incidence of dyslexia (10%), that a minimum of £368 million per annum is spent on 'unidentified dyslexics' in these sectors. This cost alone could be substantially reduced if these dyslexic individuals had been identified at an early age and provided with adequate and appropriate supportOver the last few years dyslexia has been recognised as a disability something I found hard to understand and to come to terms with my perception of disability did not include myself it is only after I truly understood the benefits and protection I could have . The definition of disability in the Disability Discrimination Act, is a physical or mental impairment which has a substantial and long-term adverse effect upon a person's ability to carry out normal day-to-day activities

SECOND-RATE CITIZENS

Is that true are we second rate citizens are we treated like other people in my opinion, there has been so many times I have been given information and expected to read and fill it in when I say I can't do it they want to help but they don't understand I am self-sufficient and can to do it myself. The worse ones for not recognising this has a disability are the Local Aurthorities, Police, Solicitors, Barristers, the scary one of all is our Government they are notorious. The dyslexic community is one of the largest minority groups in the UK if we go on 10% of the population there are millions of people who suffer with this condition but they are not aware of their Rights.

WHAT IS CLASSED AS A DISABILITY?

The definition of disability in the Disability Discrimination Act is a physical or mental impairment which has a substantial and long-term adverse effect upon a person's ability to carry out normal day-to-day activities. This includes for example:

- Sensory impairments (such as those affecting sight & hearing)

- Physical impairments (e.g. wheelchair users or someone with severe back pain)

- Specific Learning Difficulty such as dyslexia or dysphasia

- Conditions relating to mental health, such as depression, Schizophrenia, Obsessive Compulsive Disorder

- Severe facial disfigurements

- Medical conditions such as epilepsy or diabetes

Progressive medical conditions (e.g. Cancer, HIV infection and Multiple Sclerosis)

- Forms of Autism (e.g. Asperger Syndrome) Conditions which are characterised by a number of cumulative effects such as pain or fatigue (e.g. ME)

- Muscular Skeletal conditions, such as RSI, Carpal Tunnel Syndrome

- A past history of disability

ARE YOU DISABLED AS DEFINED BY THE DDA?

If you are disabled under the terms of the DDA, then this will help you to negotiate for Reasonable Adjustments in the workplace and give you legal protection if you feel you have been treated unfairly by an Employer. .

AM I DISABLED?

A recent survey showed that 52% of people who qualified as disabled under the DDA and had rights not to be treated unfairly because of their disability or health condition did not consider them disabled. People are affected by disability or health conditions in different ways. This can happen suddenly, as a result of accidents or strokes for example, or gradually as a result of conditions such as arthritis and multiple sclerosis. Some people are affected for some but not all of the time by their condition, for example people with manic depression. There is often no defining moment when a health issue becomes a disability, at least for the individual co

WHEN DOES A PERSON BECOME DISABLED?

This often depends on who is asking and the purpose of the question. Some people are classified as disabled for one purpose but not for another. The definition of disability

SHOULD I DECLARE MY DISABILITY?

Declaring a disability can sometimes be difficult for many different reasons: * you feel you will not get a job if you say you have a disability* no one can see the condition that affects you and you feel embarrassed about bringing it up* you may be worried about how your employer will respond, particularly if they have not been sympathetic to someone else in a similar situation   * you may not like asking for help because you feel you can manage or because you don't want a fuss.

* You think your manager will tell you to get on with it or tell you everyone has difficulties and they cope   * you are afraid you might lose your job because your boss will see you as less able

All of these and many more are real fears   you know your situation better than anyone else and you also know your employer. However, statistics show that one in four people either have a disability or health condition or are close to someone who does

Under the DDA, discrimination occurs where:

- a disabled person is treated less favourably than someone else

- the treatment is for a reason relating to the person's disability

- the treatment cannot be justified

In some situations, less favourable treatment may amount to "direct discrimination" and this cannot be justified.

Discrimination may also occur where:

There is a failure to make a reasonable adjustment for a disabled person
There are also measures in the DDA covering harassment and victimisation.
Under the Act discrimination also occurs when anyone knowingly aids someone to discriminate against a disabled person, or victimises anyone who tries to make use of rights under the Act.

A service provider can refuse to serve a disabled customer so long as they are able to justify such action, and their reasons have nothing to do with the customers disability and they would refuse to serve other customers in the same circumstances.

WHO IS A SERVICE PROVIDER?

All organisations that provide goods, facilities or services to the public, whether paid for or for free, are covered by the DDA, no matter how large or small they are. That includes:Hotels, guest houses, and hostels, shops, pubs and restaurants, estate agents, and private landlords, accommodation agents, councils, and housing associations, property developers, management, agencies, investment companies, and institutions, banks, and building societies, mail order, or telephone order, businesses, central and local government ,services, courts, and law firms, employment agencies, hospitals, and doctors, and dentists, clinics, churches, or other places of worship, sport and leisure facilities, bus and railway stations, amenities, and places of interest such as parks, and historic buildings, theatres and cinemas libraries and museums, telecommunications and broadcasting services.The information is available but never used I personally am discriminated against three to four times a month I receive correspondence through the post when receiving it I telephone the organisation and ask for reasonable adjustments to be made they have not got a clue what I'm talking about they are not aware of a Reasonable Adjustment in fact they usually say we have never been asked for this before and do not know what to do.The problem we face this legislation is never policed how do we police it the only way I can see it is when you're discriminated against take it through County Court the more organisations who are penalised financially it will stop them when it costs money that's when they will stop. Do we have to go to this degree I wish we didn't but I can't see any other option I have met hundreds of dyslexic people who have been destroyed by the system failed at school failed in the workplace and failed in life not enough people are aware of what these people go through if the Government understood the power of these people something will be done and if these people truly understand the power they have they will get a voice if it's going to be it is up to me.

AUGUST 2007 - DYSLEXIA A DISABILITY IN EMPLOYMENT LAW

Dyslexia can now be classed as a disability as far as employment law is concerned, following a landmark court case. It is a finding that could have a major impact on local people who suffer from the condition and the organisations that employ them."The case involved a policeman, Chief Inspector David Paterson of the Metropolitan Police Force. CI Paterson had asked for 25 per cent more time when sitting promotion exams because of his dyslexia

'REASONABLE ADJUSTMENTS.' WHAT ARE THEY?

It is the responsibility of every teacher to make reasonable adjustments. If two students have the same level of IQ and one of them has no problem with understanding and retaining information , she/he would be able to achieve his/her maximum potential in a standard classroom environment with chalk and talk delivery.Student 2, on the other hand, has major problems understanding and retaining information and is now classed as disadvantaged. The teacher has to adapt delivery of the curriculum to put it over it in a way in which student 2 can learn effectively.*If the teacher does not make those adjustments, it is classed as unlawful discrimination.* Putting the student into Special Needs does not necessarily address the problem .In some cases it can compound the problem by making the student feel stupid, and alienate him from his peers.

SO WHAT DO YOU DO?

If the student is having problems:

- Taking notes off the board. Try giving the student a printout of the information. This is a reasonable adjustment

- Problems in reading information. Use technological aids to access the information. These are reasonable adjustments.

- Persistently forgets homework, and receives detention. For a dyslexic this can be classed as unlawful discrimination. Use of a Dictaphone to record homework would be a reasonable adjustment.

WHAT DOES THAT MEAN FOR YOU?

Part 4 of the Disability Act, came into force in September 2002, offering guidance to LEAs, schools, and students, about inclusive education. The heart of the Act states that all teachers should be trained in a way that gives access to a full curriculum for all students with a disability. This includes students with Dyslexia! Teachers should also be aware of how a disability affects the student and his/her ability to learn; otherwise they can't possibly know which reasonable adjustments to make to their delivery of the curriculum. It is now essential that the Government ensures there is appropriate support for teachers, school, Collage, and universities, to help them turn the spirit of the new Act into a practical reality.

DEVELOPING THE SECRET

If I am honest I did not go out to develop internal speech I just wanted to learn how to remember spellings the problem I had faced throughout my life having problems remembering spellings I would learn a new spelling then learn another one and when I got to the fifth spelling I'd forgotten the first one all I wanted to do is retain one spelling . This is where I developed the pictorial alphabet you see Gary was a builder and you need to work with the building blocks if you can't you cannot build and Gary could not use the building blocks of literacy . This is where I realised I could not see words or letters internally and I understood you must I was a very visual person I could look at something and hold it in my mind but I couldn't with words I then realised I must make the word into a picture whch would allow me to see it the first word I learnt how to spell the word philosophy but before this point I had two get used to the building blocks letters, but my letters were pictures e.g for Apple it was the picture of an Apple that came first. I engrossed myself in internalising the information of letters, and numbers, every night before I went to sleep I would go through the alphabet in a picked form then I would go backwards from Z to A but not using pictures it must have been eight months later I was driving down the M6 motorway when all of a sudden I heard my voice in my head something that shocked me I had never heard anything before in my mind it was always silent but now I had a definite sound. Over the next few months it started to get stronger I could go all day with no sound at all and then it would start what did it sound like a whisper it was me whispering to myself .

THE DAY I LOST CONTROL

I have never had problems going to sleep at night Gary puts his head on the pillow two minutes later I'm asleep however, this night was different though, my head hit the pillow and what I discovered was what happened during the day kicked in but this time not in pictures it was with words and I could not switch off it got so bad I had to go downstairs. The next morning I asked my wife if she had ever experienced this she began to laugh yes people who have internal speech they often go through the day in their mind when they go to bed, I don't like it it kept me awake she laughed again and said welcome to my world... I was discovering new elements what I was not aware of I was developing speech "internal speech" what were the benefits, as I was doing something I began to discuss it in my mind two or three times information began to stick when people were talking to me the important issues, of what they were saying I would repeat internally and then remember them, the day I used phonics they say phonics is the way to teach, I could never use phonics untill I developed internal speech. One year ago I spelled a word internally using phonics my internal speech allowed me to manipulate the sounds internally that is the key innner speech..

CREATING THE INNER VOICE

When I first started to develop internal speech it was difficult you're creating something which you've never experienced an unknown factor. I first started with the pictorial alphabet running it through my mind there was no sound just pictorial images making sure it was in order. It took a number of months untill it felt natural to me, I was trying to make it automatic doing it without thinking once I had achieved this I progressed to stage 2 trying to create the sound as I saw the picture in my mind of an apple I created the sound of Apple I worked with the first five pictures and sound's once they were in place , I moved to the next five what does it sound like a whisper or may be quieter than a whisper very weak but once you have created all of the 26 pictures and sounds you recognise are difference it is still a whisper but with more clarity .when will I master internal speech. We have to look how long it takes to develop verbalise speech it may take 3 or 4 years it may not take this long but you have to develop it, it took Albert Einstien 3 years to develop his verbalised speech. It is developmental is it worth it? in my opinion yes.. It will help with understanding, and processing, will it help me to read? we will have to see however, there is an improvement but I'm not focusing on my reading yet I'm just developing my innerl speech and we will wait to see what happens. if we look at how a child develops using the three stages of speech development I point my attention on Vygotsky and realise one of the stages has not developed correctly inner speech this must be important for the Childs development .Since discovering the lack of my inner speech and how it is important for reading, processing, analysing, and understanding, all this affects my daughter, she struggled all the way through the primary School the Head Teacher said he had no dyslexics at the school,l there were 160 students and no dyslexics, by the age of 10 she hated school when she went to the secondary school it did not improve. Time after time myself and my wife visited the Head Teacher, and requested reasonable adjustments to be made we were refused I was taking the advice from the Disability Rights Commission, at this time but he would not make any adjustments she was a very shy inoffensive child but I could see her personality changing she was becoming angry frustrated with the education she was not getting nothing was done her anxiety levels were growing we decided to take her out of school and teach her from home .By the age of 15 she was different,t not that little shy girl any more she had had enough she had learned how to fight back, once again fight or flight and she became a fighter her problems with understanding the spoken language became a problem she had suffered with this all the way through school not understanding what the teacher said creating mass confusion if I am disciplining her I always must ask her do you understand what I'm saying. The thing is she is a bright young girl she knows it we know but the school didn't. Let's review what we have found. People with learning difficulties do not develop inner speech correctly this will have a direct influence on how they learn VISUALLY DEAF.. I can see it but cannot hear it. The lack of inner speech can affect conscience. Remember the young offenders that were discussed. Internal speech can be developed, it is speech, and speech is developmental you have to do develop it you must slow down your thoughts and learn to think linear.

I often look back through my life and wonder if it would have been any different if I had the ability to read and write correctly I am of a normal intelligence in fact I'm probably above-average would I have got good qualifications at school then go onto College and even university required a good position and life would have been a lot easier but it wasn't so Gary was born with dyslexia if I would have had one wish it would have been to be dyslexia free.

How did it happen I look at my family my Father as hidden his problems from me until now, it is only through knowing what I know now I have found he has dyslexia. My father's mother could not read could this be a genetic line and it passed down to my two children.I'm sorry if I sound bitter but you see it has been a fight all the way through my life so many times people have said Gary if you could read right and spell, you would have a good position in life they think they are paying me a complement they know I am intelligent I know I am and this is what is so frustrating. You see if I was 20 years old in 2008 I would be able to overcome my dyslexia with all the technology available however, 30 years ago it was not as recognised as is it today. As for the specialists "who by the way" may not have dyslexia, get all their information from books and studying they are able to take their qualifications however, do they really understand? it is a bit like learning how to ride a bike from of a book you can read how to ride it you can then explain about how to ride a bike but my question is can YOU ride a bike maybe not. Myself I am a dyslexic I know all the feelings and emotions dyslexic's go through all the adversities purely by experiences not through a book or studying the subject because their find it interesting being the first to find the cure..or for the university or researcher to say we have found the best way to help dyslexic's in the Educational world. This book is about dyslexia however, a dyslexic has wrote this book with the knowledge of what goes with dyslexia. The best person who has helped me is Professor Rod Nicholson because he allowed me to explain how a dyslexic feels he allowed me to do my own research on the work I had developed he is a wonderful man and I will never forget what he has done for me.. My travels all around the UK meeting the people who run the Association's to help dyslexics the British Dyslexia Association Dyslexia Action and even the   Local Dyslexia Associations what did I find them saying was that they are the voice of dyslexia but are they, one thing was clear, this area its run by females nothing against females but saying that dyslexia effects more Males than Females you would think that more males would get involved however, I have tried to get involved with them but it seems like they don't want to knw and not many of them were dyslexic in fact I never met one that was they talk of our abilities, problem-solving, thinking out of the box, but they don't let us control our own future. I've applied for many positions working in this industry and guess what? I never was successful no qualifications you see a bit ironic dont you think, they are the ones who preach about all the qualities that goes with dyslexia and having all these abilities you would think that they would receive you with open arms.

Gary all the organizations have no dyslexics at the forefront ? Yes I can only think of one or maybe two where dyslexics run it I worked with many but they would not let me in .

With the big Associations I have never met or heard of a dyslexic being at the forefront so why is that What is the solution, where do we start, maybe at the beginning when the student is in primary School we must make sure no student falls through the cracks making sure their problems have been identified and help is at hand.

When the student begins secondary school and their problems have not improved what should we do? today students are taken out of their lessons for Special Needs something I experienced myself the embarrassment this created was devastating children are cruel I remember what they said to me this is where I became unruly a problem if they said anything I just hit them but many children didn't they just said nothing and took the abuse. is this the right way to go, in my opinion NO! I have met so many people who went through the Education System struggling the emphasis was teach them how to read however, the problem with this is their education was not focused on. You must make the School aware of the child's problems if the school have not you must ask them to put in place a reasonable adjustment a few tips on reasonable adjustments… this is the problem.

1.. not to copy from the board give the child the work printed out on paper.
2 all home work to be on CD or sent by e-mail
3 always keep in touch with the your child's teacher and the teacher keeps in-touch with the parent..
4 Legislation clearly states "inclusion" yet your child's teacher allows your child to leave the class for them to go outside of the classroom for their Special Needs. Ask the child's teacher to put in-place a reasonable adjustment to prevent this "don't be fobbed off" its your child's right not to feel disadvantaged by their peers. If more parents do this the greater the awareness. Get help as soon as possible….

Dyslexia is covered by the Disability Act it says when struggling you must use alternative formats to help the student to engage with their education this might be …

ANOTHER PIECE OF THE JIGSAW

You could say now we have a dyslexic saying he has discovered what dyslexia is however, what I am saying is we have found another piece of the jigsaw puzzle which surrounds dyslexia and explains why dyslexics have the problems they do . **Am I saying dyslexia is created by the lack of inner speech yes the lack of inner speech is a major characteristic in the problems dyslexic people have. Inner speech**

is mastered by reading this helps to develop it and the person who does not master reading will not master inner speech and this is where many of their problems lie I have only given you an insight and how a dyslexic person feels.

SOLUTION

What is the solution, where do we start, maybe at the beginning when the student is in primary School we must make sure no student falls through the cracks making sure their problems have been identified and help is at hand. When the student begins secondary school and their problems have not improved what should we do? today students are taken out of their lessons for Special Needs something I experienced myself the embarrassment this created was devastating children are cruel I remember what they said to me this is where I became unruly a problem if they said anything I just hit them but many children didn't they just said nothing and took the abuse. is this the right way to go, in my opinion NO! I have met so many people who went through the Education System struggling the emphasis was teach them how to read however, the problem with this is their education was not focused on. You must make the School aware of the child's problems if the school have not you must ask them to put in place a reasonable adjustment a few tips on reasonable adjustments... this is the problem.

1.. not to copy from the board give the child the work printed out on paper.
2 all home work to be on CD or sent by e-mail
3 always keep in touch with the your child's teacher and the teacher keeps in-touch with the parent..
4 Legislation clearly states "inclusion"   yet your child's teacher allows your child to leave the class for them to go outside of the classroom for their Special Needs. Ask the child's teacher   to put in-place a reasonable adjustment to prevent this "don't be fobbed off" its your child's right not to feel disadvantaged by their peers. If more parents do this the greater the awareness. Get help as soon as possible....

Dyslexia is covered by the Disability Act it says when struggling you must use alternative formats to help the student to engage with their education this might technology, today there is technology available that allows the student to put down on paper their thoughts, you speak into the computer and words appear, other software turns text-to-speech this technology will allow the student an equal opportunity. Once the student has learnt how to use this technology they can use it throughout their lives starting with School to College University then Employment. Schools should use this technology but I know it is hard to understand but the truth is many of the students will never master reading, writing, something which teachers find hard to accept in their opinion every one can learn how to read. I do understand why they do what they do they are teachers who have been trained, and I'm sure if they truly understood the damage that they were doing they would be surprised, this is why the focus is on reading we must accept the facts and move on. When the student begins High School and Reading and Righting is a major problem you must put in-place reasonable adjustments as mentioned above... stop focusing on teaching them how to read put in soft ware that reads it to them this is not failing you are giving them an equal chance with their education.. They have this in place at Universities so how can they fail. The School starts as a stepping stone for the student to go to College, University please give them an education.

If I would have had this technology at school things Would have been a lot different for me I would have left school educated with a future maybe University I will never know.

This book has been written using this technology it has allowed me to put my thoughts on to paper a miracle for a man who left school with a reading age of seven.

Is It Right Or Wrong

in 2004 I was working in schools throughout the Midlands working with students with dyslexia I was delivering my learning programme it was successful the students enjoyed it.
I was not paid by the schools I was paid my expenses by a company named UK dyslexia live this company had invested in my programme

and were trying to make it successful.

in 2005 there was a knock on my door a tall stocky man stood there Mr Chevin I am from the Department Works and Pensions and we believe you have been working when claiming benefit I was shocked we would like you to come down to our office and make a statement . Three weeks later I attended their office they asked me questions about the work I had been doing I told them I was working with students with learning difficulties and was paid expenses I thought this would be the end of it.

Six weeks later I received a letter from Works and Pensions Solicitors saying they were taking me to Court for Fraud I could not believe it I found a solicitor and went to the Magistrates Court I explained Works and Pensions discriminated against me back in 2002 I had requested all the information on the benefit to be forwarded to me in a different format than written correspondence, they refused I contacted the Disability Rights Commission and explained the problem they decided to work on my behalf.

DISABILITY RIGHTS COMMISSION

Mr Chevin has severe dyslexia and so is unable to deal with written correspondence. Mr Chevin tells us, that he has contacted your department on a number of occasions to request that information be sent to him by audio-tape or by telephone but that you have persistently refused this request .Section 21 of the Disability Discrimination Act 1995 (DDA) places a duty on service providers to make reasonable adjustments to the way they provide a service in order to enable disabled people to access that service.After a number of months the Disability Rights Commission asked me did I want to take them to court because it was discrimination I said no. back in the Magistrates Court I was given a another time and date to appear they gave it to me in a written format I had requested an alternative format they refused at this point they have discriminated against me I lodged a complaint with their regional office after a number of weeks I received an apology.

MAGISTRATES

I understand that you are severely dyslexic and receiving the information in this format was not helpful to you. You advised Mrs Jefferies of your dyslexia and asked for the information to be sent to you by tape or email and that Mrs Smith refused to do this. I can confirm that it is not possible for information to be sent out in tape format and that the computer system that produces the hearing notices is not compatible with the email system. Having said that, it is possible for a hearing notice to be produced manually in "Word" and this could have been sent to you by email. I am disappointed that this was not offered to you by Mrs Jefferies when you explained your situation to Mrs Jefferies and I apologise for the service provided on this occasion falling below the standard that we usually expect to provide.I accepted the Magistrates apology but the problem was I pleaded Not Guilty Works and Pensions said I did not make them aware of the changes they said the Rules were in the benefit book I could not read them I told my solicitor what I had requested back in 2002 was the Rules and Regulations however, I was refused I was totally disadvantaged the solicitor didn't understand he had no knowledge on the Disability Discrimination Act my confidence in their ability was nonexistent I decided to represent myself .The prosecution offered me all the committal papers on the case I requested alternative formats they refused once again discrimination how could this be this is in the Courts of law surely they have to follow all the Rules and Regulations and laws put down for them to abide by, but they didn't, this went on for 4 months the Magistrates did not know what to do and asked for a District Judge to make a Ruling what should happen.

Dear Sir,

MAGISTRATES

I write concerning the hearing of the above matter on 12th May 2006 when the court will specifically be considering the issue regarding the format of the committal papers served on you by the Prosecution.

At the hearing on 21st April 2006 it was mentioned that this was an issue to be considered under Disability Discrimination Acts and the Criminal Procedure and Investigations Act 1996. The Legal Adviser considering the matter has brought to my attention that the issue may also involve consideration of the provisions of the Human Rights Act 1998 in particular the Right to a Fair Trial (detailed in Article 6 in Schedule 1 of that act).

I am writing to you to advise you of this in advance so that you can consider whether or not you would wish to make representations under this legislation at the hearing on 12th May 2006.

Yours faithfully,
Area Director

It wasn't only a breach of disability legislation, it was brought to my attention it was also a breach of Human Rights. It went to Crown Court I was still pleading Not Guilty I did not go out to defraud the Department of Works and Pensions I was going into school's I just wanted to help disadvantage students with my program I was not getting a income just expencies. I believed the Crown Court judge would address the Disability Discrimination and the breaches of The Human Rights Act. Surely a Crown Court judge would not allow these forms of breaches by any party . My barrister on the last moment before the case went to trial told me the prosecution had received more information this information came from the business who cked my project, when I was working with these businessmen I felt they were only doing this for financial gain I walked away they had constructed lies and fabrication about me I was grossly upset the barrister convinced me to Plead Guilty something that I did not want to do but due to the stress and anxiety I agreed.if I was given more time I could have proved these lies I asked the court to overturn my plea and brought up the breaches of disability discrimination and the breach of Human Rights Act the judge would not talk about it this was my defence he would not let me discuss these matters at all. He gave me one hour a week probation.

So now I am classed as a criminal for helping students at school this didn't seem right. I requested reasonable adjustments to be made by the probation service they agreed however, after a number of weeks they stopped sending me e-mails, I was angry now I was not going to take any more nonsense I was tired of people ignoring the legislation I make a missed judgment and get found Guilty well not again so I lodged a complaint to management one of the probation officers had discriminated against me this time from the Probation ServicesI received 8 letters of vast importance at this time I lodged a complaint with management the reply I received was not satisfactory I lodged a second complaint with higher management but once again not satisfactory I lodged my last complaint with the board over the Probation Services after two months I received a response .

PROBATION BOARD

Having dealt with those two preliminary points, the panel members then went on the address what they considered to be the subject of your complaint ie that the Probation Service had contacted you by letter on a number of occasions **after** you had specifically requested that contact should be via email. The members accepted that the facts appeared to support your complaint, and that the papers showed letters having been sent to you through the post after you had requested that communication should be done in other ways. They also accepted that you had identified your dyslexia as Reason for not wanting contact by letter, and that this was a valid reason rather than mischievous.

The members then went on to consider the National Probation Service policy on the use of emails for external contact. As you will know, the policy is generally not to use email due to concerns that:-
  a) some Courts may not accept it for evidential purposes; and
  b) Some offenders may abuse "personal" email addresses for staff by sending offensive or even threatening messages.

The panel members could therefore understand the logic behind the policy, but felt that an exception could – and should – have been made in your case given that you had identified special needs. I have therefore been asked to apologise on behalf of the service for any difficulties you may have suffered during the period that contact was undertaken by letter.After receiving the apology I decided due to the severity of discrimination, I had faced to take the matter to County Court I decided to represent myself.

I was very nervous on the morning of the hearing I had lost all faith in the English legal system after what I had experienced in Crown Court I felt it was corrupt. The case started at 10 o'clock I opened with my information covering all the aspects of discrimination I had faced the Defendant asked questions but I answered them with confidence it went on for 4 hours the Judge went away for 25 minutes then returned and said Mr Chevin you brought to my attention section 21 of the Disability Act which clearly states "Anticipatory Duties" the Probation Services did not put this place for you whilst they were serching for others methods of communication due to what they say data-protection. I believe they should have applied section 21 of the Act and clearly you have suffered discrimination and I award remedies. At last my faith returned back to the English legal system I had won but more than that it was unprecedented, it now it will help other people who have been discriminated with having dyslexia..

After winning the case I decided to take my complaint of what happed to me in the Crown Court the discrimination was un-believable and the Judge refusing to hear my defence and found me Guilty on hearing one side .of the argument its disgraceful so.

Dyslexia sufferer Gary Chevin has won a landmark legal victory after taking Staffordshire Probation Service to court for breaking disability discrimination laws.A judge at Stoke-on-Trent County Court agreed that the 49-year-old suffered discrimination when probation officers refused his request to send correspondence via email instead of letter. have taken the advice and I am taking this matter for Unlawful Discrimination and a of Human Rights Act to the European Court of Human Rights....I had never broken the law in my life accused of fraud something which I had not done faced discrimination in the Courts the Judge ignoring The Disability Act, and Breaches of the Human Rights Act that he was aware of after reading the e-mail from the Legal Department of the Lower Courts this is not Justice...

throughout this experience I suffered discrimination in the Magistrates Court, The Crown Court, the Prosecuting Solicitor, Work and Pensions, and then discrimination of the Probation Services, you would not think this area would have so much discrimination, it's the legal profession but I must be honest the worst discrimination I faced was from the prosecuting solicitor 4 months of hell I won my case with the Probation Services. with all that went on with the DWP the treatment of me was horrific this is why I am taking this to Europe . I injured my back in 1999 I tried to find employment my disability officer also tried but after many months it became nonexistent I felt useless worthless I couldn't work at the age of 40 unemployable and nobody could help me I got involved with charity work working with dyslexic people I truly understood it I did voluntary work working with students and then I developed a learning programme I thought this was my break a way to get employment the businessman who invested £170,000 but I had no contract of employment in place he said when it was successful I would get a salary but in the meantime we can only pay you expenses I believe this would lead to employment but it didn't I walked away and the businessman constructed lies saying I was paid £25,000 a year and this led to the case where I was accused of benefit fraud I wish I could change it but I can't and the discrimination I faced was unbelievable I have now got to fight against it and clear my name .

But I was not accused of fraud my charge was not making the Department of Works and pensions aware of the changes but in my defence I never had the relevant information I asked and was refused I wish I would have agreed with the disability rights commission when they asked me if I wanted to take this discrimination to court back in 1999 I was totally disadvantaged and then punished for something I did not go out to do.

ADULTS

One area which is overlooked the biggest focus is on children at school and it will be them children that will grow up and become adults and join the millions of dyslexic adults throughout the UK, how many will make the wrong decision and become figures in the prison population, and others will go through their lives unemployable not knowing what it feels like to work and produce don't get me wrong many thousands do succeed but in the bigger picture most of them don't .So what do we do? we must educate the wider world about the strengths dyslexic people have make them understand this group of people. We will be proactive in the workplace but there is a bigger problem they are now adults they have had 11 years of failing their self-esteem and self confidence is nonexistent, we must help them to regain their confidence and show them there is a future for them by opening the door to technology and helping them to develop inner speech. With the Parents I have spoken to in their opinion its an important attribute which has been overlooked for to long .So how do I see the solution? make sure self-esteem and self-confidence does not get destroyed and help us to get educated don't focus on the problem find the solution to develop the aspects what we need and allow us to develop into the people we should become, do not create crutches which are not beneficial and listen to what we say.

THE DAY UNCLE ALBERT CAME TO VISIT

It was in the mid sixties when Ian started primary school he came from a working-class family he had one brother and one sister is sister was two years older than him his brother was three years younger his father came from the Victorian beliefs and his mother was quiet and shy .Ian's sister had no problem whatsoever at school in fact academically she was top of the class everything she did came easily to her she was very protective of Ian and her younger brother Ian's younger brother also had no problems with school in fact he was reading at the age of five .Ian's father was a proud quiet man he demanded discipline from his children just a look was enough when he looked at you it sent shivers running through your spine nobody answered him back he worked as a milkman getting up very early in the morning working seven days a week .Ian's mother worked in the local industry she waited on his father like a maid she never answered him back he was the king of the house.After 18 months in the primary School Ian's teacher approached his mother. Mrs Davies we think Ian has a problem he is not advancing with his reading we think he needs to be tested. That night Ian's mother tried to explain to his father what the teacher had said about his reading his father said if he can't read so what he doesn't need reading to work in a factory and that's the only thing his father said on the matter

Months past Ian was feeling the pressure he knew something was not right all his friends could now read easily but he could not is confusion was growing but his self belief was decreasing. It was late summer when Ian bought home a letter from school he gave it to his mother it was an appointment it was to meet a Child Psychologist the letter asked for two signatures and could they attend Ian's mother signed it but she never asked his father. Two months later Ian and his mother went for the appointment Mrs Edwards was a pleasant lady with a really nice smile she told him to sit down with his mother she explained they were going to do a number of tests it took probably one hour to complete, at the end she told his mother they would get the results in about six weeks. Ian's mother never told his father about the test then one day Ian brought another letter home it was from his teacher asking his mother to come into school , next Friday at 3:30 p.m. Ian and his mother went to school they met Mrs Jackson come and sit down she said with a strange look on her face we have had the results what are they Ian's mother said, Ian has dyslexia a look of panic appeared on his mother's face dyslexia what is that can it be cured can the doctors help him will he have to take medication she started to cry I knew Ian would have something wrong with him she said, Mrs Jackson tried to console Ian's mother, it is not that bad she said there is something we can do to help him. That evening Ian's mother decided to tell his father dyslexia what is that just another posh name for somebody who is a dunce they come out with all these special names it's rubbish my son is just a bit thick . It was getting harder for Ian he was not improving in fact, it was getting worse he was a very quiet shy boy with only one friend. At playtime all the boys had magazines with footballers in them they used to swap the cards but Ian had never read one magazine in his life once again he could not take part in something boys did he was getting very upset every night he would cry into his pillow begging God to help him please God help me I don't want to be a dunce help me to be cleverer help me to read. This went on for a number of years crying in his bed alone nobody knew about this and the damage it was doing. Ian's mother and father never discussed Ian's dyslexia it was never mentioned his father would say well he's not that bright but you don't have to be bright to work in a factory his future had been sorted out by his father...Ian was now 12 years of age school had been terrible so far but now he was going to the secondary school. If he thought it had been bad so far it was going to get worse in this place there was no time for people who could not read you are just a dunce and nobody had the time to help Ian hated it and the other students were terrible, children zoom in on people's weaknesses and that's what they did dunce, dummy, stupid, the names they called him he can't read never mind he is simple. Ian's self-esteem was now rock bottom he still went to bed at night and cried into his pillar but did not pray to God anymore he felt that God had forgotten him it got so bad Ian considered suicide. He was now 14 years of age nobody knew what he was going through. It was early January a new teacher had come to the school Mr Tavern he was the physics teacher sit down and be quiet he said Ian was at the back of the class a place where he always sat nobody could see him here he would blend in the background today's lesson is on Albert Einstein the most smartest man who ever walked the earth Mr Tavern, explained to the class what Einstein had done how he had changed the world Ian was amazed. That night he thought why couldn't I be like Albert Einstein why couldn't I have been born like him Ian became fascinated with Einstein one Saturday Ian was walking through the local market when he saw a poster of Albert Einstein pulling a funny face how much is that poster he said one pound he brought it Ian went home; clutching the poster in his hand ran to his room and put it on the wall.Another bad day at school Ian went home went straight upstairs and lay on his bed he looked up at Einstein began to talk to him, Uncle Albert I have had a terrible day I wish I was like you I would give anything for this, over the next few months Ian did not seem so bad because he has found a new friend who listens to him he listens to all the problems he has at school uncle Albert listens to them and never judges him.Ian was now in his last year at school the Monday morning Jane came Jane was a new teacher but she was different very young just out of university Ian liked her at the end of the class can Ian stay behind she said, sit-down Ian I want to talk to you I'm a special teacher I help people with your kind of problems she asked Ian what he liked Ian told her about Albert Einstein she smiled you don't know do you, what said Ian, I don't know what your talking about Einstein what about Einstein, he was dyslexic, Ian could have fell off his chair he did not say anything Einstein had problems at school he was dyslexic she said again he was just like you Ian couldn't believe it Uncle Albert like me. Ian went home he wen straight upstairs and lay on his bed staring at Uncle Alber From the moment Jane told him about uncle Albert something changed in side of Ian if Uncle Albert could do it why can't I we are both the same we are both dyslexic Ian's self-limiting believes began to break away and in his heart he felt maybe I can succeed . Wednesday morning, Ian went to find Jane can you help me he said, yes of cause I can Ian, the examination are coming up next month I want to pass, then what have you got in mind, she said could you read me the questions and then I could give you the answer, well I must ask the Head Teacher it was agreed Ian could answer the questions and Jane could write them .

THE RESULTS

Ian was given his results he came top in everything for the first time in his life he had come first the other students said it was a fake but Ian knew it wasn't he always knew he was the smartest but could never prove it .Ian now had a different outlook on life yes he still struggled but he now believed anything was possible if Uncle Albert could achieve what he did with all of the problems he faced as a dyslexic so could Ian he now believed anything is possible THANK YOU UNCAL ALBERT....

Gary how do you feel you have finished your first book over 40,000 words ? Something I never thought I would do it was an impossibility to me 10 years ago I thank prof Nicholson it is his fault he suggested to me to write the book but since I've started I now cannot stop I have another book running through my mind .

Gary Chevin 28. 10 .2007

LaVergne, TN USA
14 December 2009

166953LV00004B/122/P